Speaking of
SKIN CARE

This book tells you how to look younger and more beautiful. By simply taking care of your skin which, exposed to all kinds of weather conditions, day and night, needs constant attention. It covers in an informative manner such topics as common skin infections and their remedies, massage and ageing, facials and packs, and use of cosmetics for makeup. It also tells you how to avoid, control and treat skin diseases, which are described at length, with a little effort on your own part and some advice by your family doctor.

A well-known cosmetologist and one of the pioneers of beauty therapy in India, Parvesh Handa opened a beauty clinic in New Delhi in 1977 and another in Chandigarh in 1980. She has written several books on beauty care and contributed articles to newspapers and magazines.

Other titles in Health and Cure Series

Ayurvedic Herbal Cures
Yoga—A Practical Guide
Yoga and Nature Cure Therapy
Stress Management through Yoga & Meditation
Heart Care: Lifestyle & Longevity
Body, Mind and Soul: The Complete Beauty Book
Ayurvedic Remedies for Common Diseases
Alternative Medicine Acupuncture
Nature Cure
Stress: An Owner's Manual
Overcoming Anxiety
First Aid for Animals
Heart Attacks
Fitness Over 40
The Pregnant Year
Child Care
Sleeping Problems
Diabetes and Diet
High Blood Pressure
You and Your Medicines
Healing Through Gems
Oriental Stories as Tools in Psychotherapy
Positive Family Therapy
Psychotherapy of Everyday Life

**Published by
Sterling Publishers Private Limited**

Speaking of
SKIN CARE

PARVESH HANDA

A Sterling Paperback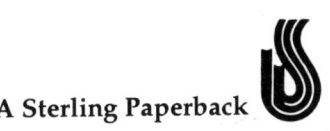

STERLING PAPERBACKS
An imprint of
Sterling Publishers (P) Ltd.
A-59, Okhla Industrial Area, Phase-II,
New Delhi-110020.
Tel: 26387070, 26386165; Fax: 91-11-26383788
E-mail: info@sterlingpublishers.com
www.sterlingpublishers.com

Speaking of Skin Care
© 1998, Parvesh Handa
ISBN 978-81-207-1944-6
Fourth Reprint 2005
Fifth Reprint 2008

All rights are reserved. No part of this publication
may be reproduced, stored in a retrieval system or transmitted,
in any form or by any means, mechanical, photocopying,
recording or otherwise, without prior written permission
of the original publishers.

Published by Sterling Publishers (P) Ltd., New Delhi-110020.
Printed at Sterling Publishers Pvt. Ltd., New Delhi-110020.

PREFACE

Every woman wants to be beautiful. But while some are born beautiful, others are not. Those who are born beautiful may look worn out with the pasage of time. This is the reason why, in order to stay beautiful, women of all ages need expert advice—commonly known as "Beauty Care". Indeed, skin care is essential for not only women but also men, for the prolongation of youthful looks.

Beauty products were invented to enhance natural beauty and it is very important that a woman should know that what are various skin disorders or diseases which mar beauty and which kind of creams and lotions should be used to keep the skin free of blemishes. Everyone covets that natural but beautiful look with healthy glowing skin—and for achieving that, one has to work internally as well as externally, with a little help from nature and with the art of skilful make-ups. But before starting anything, it is imperative that you take a look at the skin—the largest organ of the human body which is as hard working as your heart or lungs.

I always advise my reader to go for natural preventives, herbal treatments and home-made remedies. These home-made preparations are effective to maintain beauty of skin without any side-effects. In case of serious problems these potions act as a soothing back-up, but it is always advisable to consult a doctor. I am grateful to Dr. Jitender Arora, M.B.B.S., M.D., Head of the Department of Skin and V.D., Medical College; and Associated Hospitals, Jammu who have assisted me in writing a few chapters on dermatology. I hope this book will reveal how common skin problems and diseases can be avoided, controlled or cured with a little effort on your part, and where necessary, a bit of guidance from the family doctor.

While planning for the book, the intention was to make it easily comprehensible and readable for the common reader. To this effect the language has been specifically kept simple, easy and lucid with relevant illustrations. Thanks to the amazing advances in medical sciences, the discomforts connected with the skin diseases have become much easier to cope with.

It is generally seen that the commonest problems of the skin are excessive dryness or oiliness, enlarged pores, muddy look, blemishes and blackheads, etc. These are caused by internal disorders, an improper diet, insufficient rest, lack of fresh air and exercise and above all, indifferent skin cleansing habits. Remember, good eating habits as well as correct selection and use of proper cosmetics can correct all these probelms. If you are in search of a smooth complexion, maintain healthy habits with a healthy appetite.

When a woman is hot, angry or embarrassed, her skin changes colour from pink to red. When she is tired and upset, her skin looks puffy and pale. The skin blooms with dewy freshness, when it is young, it wrinkles and dries out with age. This book tells how to look younger and more beautiful. Your skin, which is exposed to all kinds of weather conditions, needs constant attention.

I would welcome suggestions for the improvement of this volume.

Parvesh Handa

CONTENTS

Preface v

1. **Study of Skin and Scalp**   1
   - Historiology of the Skin
   - Types of Skin
   - Caring for the Skin
   - Effect of Natural Sources on Skin
   - Diet and Your Skin
   - Role of Minerals for Beauty

2. **Skin Afflictions**   12
   - Lesions
   - Common Skin Diseases
   - Lumps and Bumps - The Skins Imperfections

3. **Skin Diseases**   33
   - Treatment of Pimples
   - Acne and Its Cure
   - Warts on the Face
   - Contagious Diseases of the Skin: Scabies
   - Thrush (Candida)
   - Skin Inflammations
   - Urticaria
   - Psoriasis
   - Leucoderma—The Whitening of Skin
   - Leprosy
   - Infection of Red Swelling of the Nail-fold and between Fingers
   - White Marks on Fingernails
   - Rough, Tired and Itchy Feet

4. **Caring for the Skin** — 51
   - Hormones and Their Effect on the Skin
   - Caring for the Skin by Electric Therapy
   - Light Therapy
   - Quick Home Facials
   - Skin Care by Reflex Therapy
   - Skin Surgery
   - Baby's Skin Care
   - Oils and Your Skin

5. **Body Odour** — 62
   - Vaginal Odour: Causes and Cures
   - Sweating Excessively
   - Baths for Skin Care
   - Breathing and Exercises
   - Cleanliness
   - How to Bathe

6. **Premature Ageing** — 69
   - Physiological Effects of Massage
   - For a Bulging Bottom

7. **Hirsutism** — 75
   - Can Medicines help reduce Hairiness
   - What to do for Excessive Hair on Face and Body
   - What is Hirsutism and what are Its Causes?
   - How does one get rid of Superfluous Hair Cosmetically?
   - Precautions for Using Electrical Devices

8. **Healthy Hair** — 83
   - Home-made Herbal Hair Tonic
   - Baldness among Men and Women
   - Dandruff
   - Patchy Baldness
   - Greying of Hair
   - Dry, Brittle and Dull Hair
   - Hair Conditioning
   - Pediculosis—Lice Infestation

9. **Beauty of the Breasts** — 93
   - Do not neglect Your Breasts
   - Supporting Your Breasts

- How to measure the Cups
- How to choose a Bra
- Breast Care for Lactating Mothers
- Abdominoplasty—Body Contouring

10. **Common Conditions of Genitalia**   **99**
    - Genital Scabies
    - Genital Warts
    - Genital Herpes
    - Candidiasis or Moniliasis
    - Phimosis and Aids Virus
    - Tumours of the Skin
    - Difference between Skin Cancer and Tumours
    - Cystitis

1
STUDY OF SKIN AND SCALP

The skin is the largest organ in the human body and is composed of cells which keep dying but are being renewed all the time. Indeed, skin care is essential for the prolongation of youthful looks, not only for women but also for men. With a little care, skin problems and diseases can be avoided, controlled or cured.

A healthy skin is characterised by slight moisture, softness, flexibility, a slightly acidic reaction and the absence of any blemish or disease. It must possess a smooth, fine-grained texture, be affirmable visually and by touch. The skin of the scalp is essentially similar to the skin found elsewhere on the human body, except for the larger and deeper hair follicles which are present on the scalp for accommodating longer hair.

Historiology of the Skin

The skin's surface is not made up of just one single layer. It has two defined layers — the epidermis and the dermis. The epidermis, also called the scarf skin, is the outermost layer of the skin which provides a protective covering for the inner layer and contains no blood vessels but has many small nerve endings.

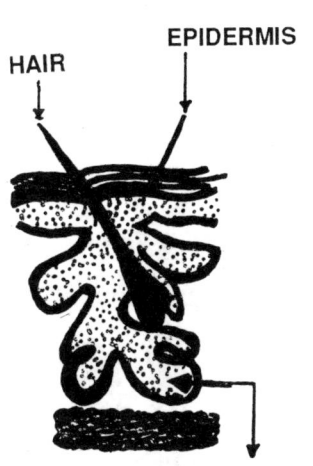

Body hair and follicle

The dermis, which is the inner layer of the skin, is also known as derma, carium, cutis or true skin. The dermis is highly sensitive and is a vascular layer of connective tissues containing numerous blood vessels, lymph vessels, nerves, sweat glands, oil glands, hair follicles and muscles. The dermis itself consists of two layers — the papillary or superficial layer and reticular or deeper layer. The skin receives its nourishment from the blood and lymph. Between half and two-thirds of the total blood supply of the body is distributed to the skin which contains numerous capillaries. The blood and the lymph circulating through the skin contribute to its growth and nourishment. The skin contains the surface endings of many nerve fibres, classified as follows:

1) Motor nerve fibres which are distributed to the blood vessels and the arrector pipli muscles of the hair follicles.
2) Sensory nerve fibres which react to heat, cold, touch, pressure and pain.
3) Secretory nerve fibres which are distributed to the sweat and oil glands of the skin.

The pliability of the skin depends upon the elasticity of the fibres of the dermis. When a healthy skin expands, it regains its former shape immediately, whereas an aged skin, on the other

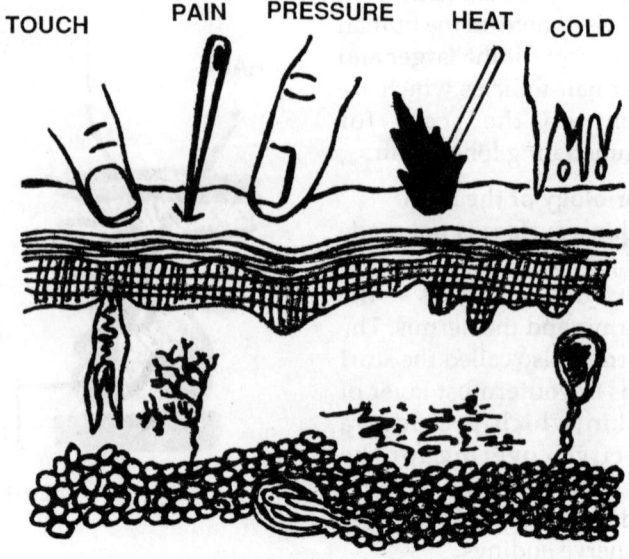

Sensory nerves of the skin

hand, is characterised by its loss of elasticity. The complexion depends primarily upon the melanin or colouring matter deposited in the stratum and the papillary layer of the dermis and partly on the blood supply in the skin.

Cleanliness keeps the skin free from blemishes. The skin contains two types of duct glands which extract materials from the blood to form new substances. The first type is known as the sweat gland which secretes sweat. The other type is the sebaceous or oil gland which secretes sebum — a semi-fluid oily substance flowing through the oil ducts. However, when the sebum becomes hardened and the ducts are blocked, a blackhead is formed.

Types of Skin
Normally, your skin will fall into one of the categories of Normal, Dry and Greasy. If the skin feels smooth, supple and elastic, it is normal. A healthy, normal skin is unblemished, velvety, smooth and supple, with no enlarged pores or flaky dead cells. A flaky and dull skin is generally dry with a tendency towards broken veins, flakiness and dry patches, and it needs a lot of care. If neglected, it turns into wrinkles and lines. A greasy skin often has blackheads and is prone to acne and several disorders which shall be discussed later on in detail.

Most people have a combination skin. In this type of skin, the middle of the face (patches on the forehead, nose and the chin) is shiny with a dilated and coarse texture. The rest of the face has either normal or dry skin.

Blackheads, whiteheads, steatoma, asteatosis, sebarrhoea, pimples, acne vulgaris, bromidrosis (osmidrosis), anidrosis, hyderidrosis, prickly heat, sunburn, inflammations, dermititis, eczema, ringworm, red veins, lesions, leucoderma, leprosy, burns and scalds, freckles, birthmarks and scars, wrinkles, hirsutism, warts, moles, scabies, boils, blotchiness, odour and fungus infection, psoriasis, double chin, melasma, thrush (candidal), scabies, sycosis barbac, chronic paronychie, intertrigo, herpes, urticaria, skin tumours, photodermatitis, lichen planus, erytheme mutliforme are some of the chronic disorders and allergies which mar many a lovely face. These serious skin problems will be discussed in much detail with suitable remedies by cosmetology or by herbal treatment.

skin — cross-section

Labels: Epidermis, Dermis, Sweat pore, Sebaceous gland, Sweat tube, Touch corplegle, Sweat gland, Root of hair, Fat cells

Caring for the Skin

The sun, cold, rain, heat, wind and water all are natural phenomena which can affect the skin. The effects can be favourable or adverse. The condition of the skin varies with the weather. During winter, it tends to become dry and should be treated as such. In summer, the skin generally becomes oily. Hence, skin care should be adapted to the change in climate. The following summary should help:

Summer Care
1) Wash the face with soap at least twice a day.
2) Cleanse the skin thoroughly before going to bed at night.
3) Apply astringent lotion on an excessive oily skin.
4) Wash the face and bathe with cold water.
5) Perform a home facial once a week.

Winter Care
1) Avoid using soap as far as possible.
2) Clean the face before going to bed and remove the accumulated dirt and cosmetics on the skin.
3) Wash the face once a day, using tepid water.
4) Perform a home facial once a fortnight.

5) Apply a rich cream and moisturiser at night and also when going out in cold and dry weather.
6) If your skin is excessively dry, application of a vitaminised face cream at night is recommended.

Monsoon Care
1) A three-step skin care programme in cleansing, toning and moisturising should be made part of your daily routine.
2) Do not forget that an oily skin needs a moisturiser too. Lack of moisture enhances the tell-tale lines, giving an impression of older age.
3) Moisturise the area around your eyes daily at night. Wipe off the excess cream after 30 minutes. This will ensure that your eyes are not puffy the next morning.
4) Steam the face at least once a week if your skin is blemished. Clean the face thoroughly before steaming to unclog the pores of the skin.

Effect of Natural Sources on Skin

The sun, cold, rain, heat and water certainly have an effect on the skin.

Sun

It clears the skin of acne, heals mild infections, cleanses oily skins, gives a lovely tan and revives the whole body. On the other hand, the heat of the sun can wither a dry skin, burn a delicate one, distend the veins and cause burns and sunstroke. Sunbathing must be progressive, beginning with a few minutes on the first couple of days, ten minutes the next few days, fifteen minutes after a week and so on, as far as you may comfortably bear its duration.

Remember the following points:
1) Never expose yourself continuously to strong sunrays for more than half an hour.
2) Ensure that sunrays affect the whole surface of your body, instead of affecting only one side. Playing, walking or swimming in the sunlight is the best way.
3) Oil your skin generously, unless you have a naturally greasy skin.
4) Wear a hat and protect your eyes with sun-glasses.

5) Do not use eau-de-Cologne, perfume or deodorants as they often contain ingredients which can cause brown marks and irritation to the skin.
6) Do not wear heavy make-up. Lipstick changes colour and mascara runs.
7) Watch carefully the most exposed parts of the body, lest sunburn occurs. Put plenty of oil on these parts of the body and cover them at the first sign of reddening.

The Cold

Cold roughens the skin, particularly the dry and sensitive types. It makes the skin dry, cracks the skin and hinders the blood circulation. Protect you skin with a thick coating of cream. Even an oily skin must be lubricated during winter. Use an oily cream or cocoa-butter on your lips. Avoid going abruptly from the cold outside to a hot air-conditioned room as this can cause blood vessels under the skin to burst and may give you a blotchy complexion. Sudden exposure to intense cold can produce blotchiness, hasten the appearance of thread veins on the cheeks and other sensitive parts and give the skin a flaky appearance.

Rain

Rain water is good for every type of skin. Do not hesitate to expose your face to the rain. Protect your hair with a water-proof covering.

The Heat

Heat has a drying, ageing effect on all but the most oily of skins. As the natural oils begin to dry, the skin becomes leathery and may wrinkle. The leathery texture and brown pigment are actually the skin's own natural protections against the effect of ultraviolet radiation. As extra Vitamin D is produced in the skin when the body is exposed to radiation, the skin produces melanin, the brown pigment, to protect itself against excessive production of Vitamin D and to prevent sunburn.

The great merit of heat is that it makes you perspire, thereby eliminating a great quantity of toxic matter and cleansing the pores of the skin. Drink plenty of liquid and eat more salt than usual, as perspiration brings out a great deal of water and mineral salts. Wear light, loose clothes and change your underwear daily. Another important factor has been discovered that can help to solve the problem of burning the skin. The level of Vitamin A in the blood drops after the body is exposed to intensive ultraviolet radiation, so taking extra Vitamin A just before and during a holiday helps to prevent burning by increasing the thickness of the skin. Stores of Vitamin A in the body are affected too by the extra Vitamin D formed during exposure to the sun. Consequently, taking extra Vitamin A helps to restore the natural balance. The level of Vitamin A in the body drops during menstruation, so extra care is needed if you sunbathe at this time. Remember, never sunbathe between 12 noon and 2 p.m.

Wind
The wind stimulates the circulation and can be a tonic to the system but it dries the skin, especially during winter. When you go out in cold or strong wind, protect your facial skin with a good coating of cold cream.

Water
Tap water can be good for your skin depending on your skin type and the hardness or softness of water. If your skin is extremely dry, washing your face with tap water will not be helpful, for the presence of salts and calcium in the water will almost certainly be drying.

Do and Don'ts
1) Use water-softeners. It will help to counteract this effect. However, it is more practical to use softening substances, such as a bath salt or oil for bathing the body.
2) Beware of using hard water on your face.
   Many beauty specialists recommend sea water baths for the skin. Sea water cleanses the skin, firms the muscles, stimulates the circulation and tones up the body.
3) After having a swim or bath in sea water, wash yourself with fresh water.
4) Rub a little almond oil on the skin after having a bath in the sea, and then splash with fresh water.
5) When you swim in sea water, protect your hair with a water-tight cap.

Diet and Your Skin

For a blemish-free, sparkling skin, you must keep in mind the following five points:
1) Eat wisely.
2) Take plenty of rest.

3) Learn proper breathing.
4) Keep your body supple.
5) Observe cleanliness.

The skin must be constantly renewed to remain healthy. This means that cell movement must be encouraged by good circulation. Vitamin C purifies and vitalises the bloodstream. It is found in citrus fruits like orange, lemon and grapefruit. Green vegetables and potatoes also contain Vitamin C. The important point here is that Vitamin C cannot be stored by the body and so must be supplied daily.

For healthy formation, the skin also needs Vitamin B_2 from fresh vegetables, milk and wholewheat. Alcohol, coffee and tea interfere with the body's ability to assimilate Vitamin B. If you replace them by unsweetened orange or grapefruit juice, you are doing your skin a good service. Diet is a widely discussed subject—what to eat and what not to eat. It is advised that you must eat a little of everything.

Do's
1) Eating at regular hours helps the intestines to function properly and as a result clears the complexion.
2) Always prefer fresh to canned food.
3) Drink a lot of water (five to six glasses a day) to eliminate the toxins from your blood.
4) Don't eat a heavy lunch as it makes one sleepy. Enjoy a substantial meal in the evening in a relaxed atmosphere, such as an hour before you go to bed so that the digestive process is completed.
5) Eat slowly and cheerfully.

Dont's
1) Avoid fried and greasy foods, sweets and alcohol. They can cause blemishes and blotchiness.
2) Beware of raw meat, starchy foods and alcoholic drinks, which are the natural enemies of your liver and your skin.

Rest
The conditions of life are exhausting in the present-day world. Life has brought more responsibilities, duties and worries. You must sleep at least eight hours every night and more than eight hours when feeling run down. Therefore, a third of your life should be spent in bed for complete rest.

Study of Skin and Scalp

You must relax occasionally during the day to restore your energy. Try the Hollywood "Beauty Angel". Lie on the floor on your back and put the feet up on a chair. Stay in this position for a few minutes as this will send the blood to your head and increase the blood supply to the scalp. Do not stay in the "Beauty Angel" position for more than 20 minutes in a day.

Do's
1) Do not read in bed, but if you must, then read a boring book.
2) Relax completely in bed. Normal sleep is very essential for a healthy complexion.
3) Avoid anything which might excite or stimulate you, such as noisy entertainment, arguments, use of alcohol and tobacco.
4) Before going to bed, wash in warm water and take a warm soothing drink.
5) When you wake up after a sound sleep, allow yourself five minutes to stretch.

Dont's
1) Avoid taking sleeping pills and tranquillisers.
2) Do not drink tea or coffee after 6 p.m. Have a light dinner.
3) Take a quiet walk before going to bed.

Caloric Values of Indian Foods and Drinks

a) **Nuts per 100 gms** — *Calories*

Almond	655
Dry Coconut	662
Groundnut	567
Walnut	687
Pistachio Nut	626

b) **Dairy Products per 100 gms**

Milk [Buffalo's]	117
Milk [Cow's]	120
Butter	729
Ghee	900

c) **Fruits per 100 gms**

Banana	116
Cherries	64
Dates	317

Mango	:	74
Melon	:	17
Organge	:	48
Papaya	:	32
Grapes	:	58
Guava	:	51
Sweet Lemon	:	35
Apple	:	19
Apricot	:	53

d) **Non-Vegetarian -100 gms**

Fish	:	111
Prawn	:	89
Egg	:	173
Goat Meat	:	118

e) **Drinks**

Water	:	No calories	
Black Coffee	:	Negligible	
Black Tea	:	Negligible	
Jaljeera	:	Less than 10	
Lemon Squash	:	18	
A Cup of Tea	:	22	(without sugar)
A Cup of Tea	:	78	(with sugar)
Tomato Juice	:	25	
Orange Juice	:	36	
Rose Syrup	:	47	
Pine Apple Juice	:	65	
Milk, one glass	:	175	
Skimmed Milk	:	130	
Red Wine	:	100	
Brandy [1 peg]	:	75	
Whisky [1 peg]	:	88	
Beer [1 glass]	:	144	

Role of Minerals for Beauty

Like vitamins, minerals are also required in very small quantities in our food. There are about 20 minerals, most of which are present in minute quantities in the body. Most of you must be knowing the functions of these minerals. Iron and calcium are the important minerals and require most consideration while selecting diets. If our food intake provides the recommended amount of these two minerals, our needs for the other minerals are met.

Iron
The amount of iron present in our body is very small but it is very vital to our health. Blood cells contain a substance called haemoglobin, the red colouring matter of the blood cells, which in turn contains iron. These red blood cells are the carriers of oxygen from the lungs to the tissues, and carbon dioxide from the tissues to the lungs. During the performance of this function, these blood cells wear out and are then broken down by the liver. The iron from them is reused in the formation of fresh haemoglobin.

Iron is also stored in almost all body tissues, in the liver, spleen and bone marrow. Once the body has sufficient iron, the question of whether we need more iron in our daily diet arises. The answer is yes. Dietary iron must be supplied to compensate for daily loss through excretion and during the period of menstruation for women. Iron is, therefore, important because it is an essential element of both blood and muscle haemoglobin and is important for the prevention of nutritional anemia — a condition in which there is a reduction of the number of red blood cells or haemoglobin in the bloodstream which causes a depletion of vigour and energy.

Calcium
It is the most abundant mineral element in the body. An adult man weighing about 55 to 60 kgs would have approximately 950 gms. of calcium in the body. Out of this amount, over 95 per cent calcium of the body is found in the bones and teeth while the balance is in the blood and body fluids. Calcium is needed by all age groups. Small losses of calcium occur daily in the body's waste products. Calcium levels of the blood and the body fluids must be maintained. When the calcium intake in the body is insufficient, calcium is drawn out of the bones to meet the blood and the body fluid requirements. This is the reason why older people usually have fragile bones as a result of the withdrawal of bone calcium to meet blood and body fluid needs. Calcium requirements also increase during pregnancy and nursing mothers require increased calcium, not only to meet their own requirements but also for milk production in the body.

2
SKIN AFFLICTIONS

Lesions
A lesion is a structural change in the tissues caused by injury or disease. These are of two types: primary and secondary.

Primary Lesions
1) *Macule* : A small discoloured spot or patch on the surface of the skin, neither raised nor sunken.
2) *Papule* : A small elevated pimple on the skin containing no fluid, but which may develop pus.
3) *Wheal* : An itchy, swollen spot that lasts only for a few hours. This is usually caused by mosquito or insect bites.

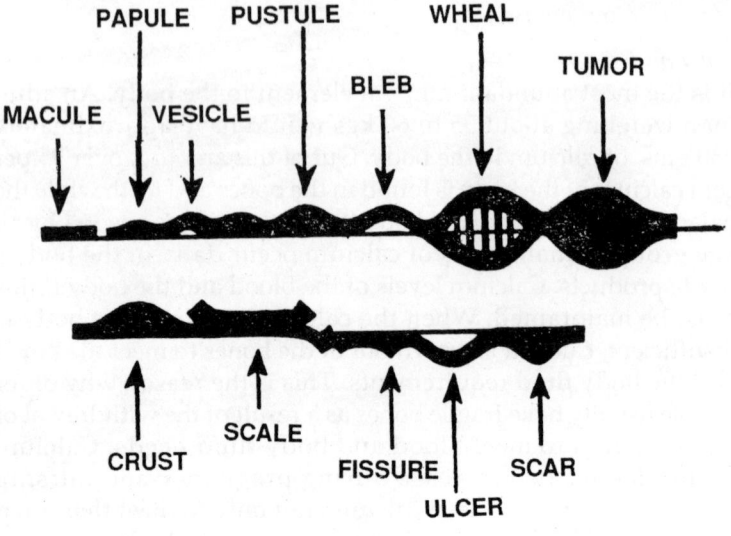

Skin lesions

Skin Afflictions

4) *Tubercle* : A soiled lump larger than a papule, which projects above the surface of the skin or lies within or under the skin, varying in size from a pea to a nut.
5) *Tumour* : An external swelling, varying in size, shape and colour.
6) *Vesicle* : A blister with clear fluid in it. It lies just beneath the epidermis and is smaller in size.
7) *Bulla* : A blister containing watery fluid. It is similar to a vesicle but larger in size.
8) *Pustule* : An elevation of the skin with an inflamed base and which contains pus. It looks like a common pimple.

Secondary Lesions

The secondary lesions are those skin diseases which develop in the later stages and are of a serious nature. These are:

1) *Scale* : An accumulation of the epidermal flakes. It may be dry or greasy.
2) *Crust* (Scab) : An accumulation of sebum and pus, mixed, perhaps, with the epidermal material.
3) *Excoriation* : A skin abrasion produced by scratching or scraping. It may be due to the loss of superficial skin after an injury.
4) *Fissure* : A crack in the skin penetrating into the derma as in the case of a chapped skin.
5) *Ulcer* : An open lesion on the skin or mucous membrane of the body, accompanied by pus and loss of skin depth.
6) *Scar* : It is likely to form after the healing of an injury or skin condition that has penetrated the dermal layer.
7) *Stain* : An abnormal discoloration of the skin.

Common Skin Diseases

A disease is any departure from a normal state of health. A skin disease is an infection of the skin which is visible and may consist of scales, pimples or pustules. Some of the common terms applied to skin diseases are:

1) *An acute disease* : is manifested by symptoms of a more or less violent character and is of a short duration.
2) *A chronic disease* : is of long duration, usually mild but recurring.
3) *An infectious disease* : is caused by pathogenic germs taken into the body as a result of contact with a contaminated object.

4) *A contagious disease* : is communicable by contact.
5) *A congenital disease* : is one that is present in the infant at the time of birth.
6) *A seasonal disease* : is influenced by the weather, like rashes caused by prickly heat in summer.
7) *An occupational disease* : is afflicted by one's occupation.
8) *A parasitic disease* : is one that is caused by a vegetable or an animal parasite, such as pediculosis or ringworm.
9) *A pathogenic disease* : is produced by a disease-producing bacteria.
10) *A systemic disease* : is the result of overfunctioning of the internal glands and is caused by a faulty diet.
11) *A venereal disease* : is a contagious disease commonly acquired by contact with an infected person during sexual intercourse.
12) *An epidemic disease* : is the manifestation of the disease that attacks simultaneously a large number of persons living in a particular locality.
13) *An allergy*: is a sensitivity which certain persons develop due to normally harmless substances. Skin allergies are very common and are caused by contact with certain types of foods, cosmetics, medicines and tints. This may result in itching, accompanied by redness, swelling, blisters, oozing and scaling. An inflammation is characterised by redness, pain, swelling and heat.

Sebaceous Gland Diseases
1) *Blackheads* : These are a worm-like mass of hardened sebum, appearing most frequently on the face, forehead

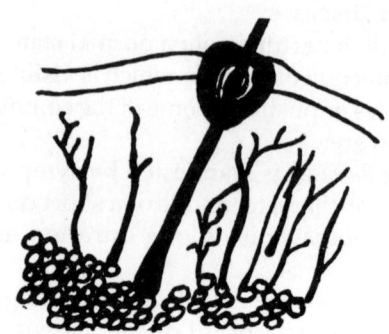

Blackhead forming around the mouth of a hair follicle

and the nose. Blackheads always accompany pimples and often occur during the teens.
2) *Whiteheads (Milia)*: These are caused by the accumulation of sebaceous matter beneath the skin. They occur on different parts of the face, neck, chest and the shoulders. Whiteheads are usually associated with fine textured and often dry skin.
3) *Steatoma (Sebaceous cyst)* : It is a subcutaneous tumour of the sebaceous glands filled with sebum, varying in shape from the size of a pea to that of an orange. It usually occurs on the scalp, neck and the back.
4) *Asteatosis* : It is a condition of dry scaly skin characterised by absolute or relative deficiency of sebum, due to senile changes or some bodily disorders. It generally develops in old age; in youth it may be caused by the reaction of alkalies such as soaps and washing powders.
5) *Seborrhoea* : It is a skin condition due to overactivity and excessive secretion of the sebaceous or oil glands. An itching or burning sensation may accompany it. An oily condition or shining of the nose, forehead, or scalp indicates the presence of seborrhoea.
6) *Acne* : It is a chronic inflammatory disease occurring most frequently on the face, back and the chest. Acne appears in a variety of forms ranging from simple non-contagious pimples to a serious deep-seated skin condition.

Sweat Gland Diseases
1) *Bromidrosis or Osmidrosis* : It refers to foul smelling perspiration, usually noticeable in the armpits or on the feet.
2) *Anidrosis* : It refers to lack of perspiration (consult a doctor)
3) *Hyderidrosis* : It refers to excessive perspiration and is caused by excessive heat or body weakness (consult a doctor)
4) *Miliaria rubra (Prickly heat)* : It is generally caused by exposure to excessive heat and is accompanied by burning and itching of the skin.

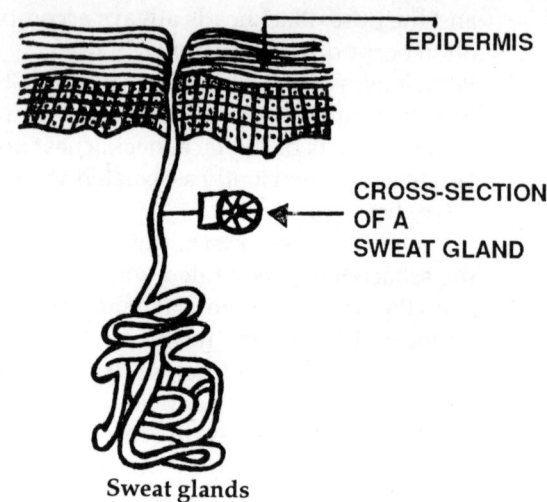
Sweat glands

Lumps and Bumps : The Skin Imperfections
Any kind of spot on the face spoils the appearance of a woman. Every beauty-conscious woman wants to avoid such beauty-deterrents. Spots are of various kinds like black spots beneath the eyes, white patches, smallpox spots (pock marks), burns and scalds, discoloration of the skin, sunburn, birthmarks, freckles, cracked skin, prickly heat, red veins on the cheeks, boils and pustules, blotchiness, bruises and wounds, chilbrow, whitlow, guinea worm, pigmentation and cold sores.

Lines around the Eyes
These are among the first to form on the face but they are not caused only by age. They are caused by expressions as much as anything and as such are known as "Laughter lines". These fine, upward slanting laughter lines are attractive and give character to a face. The downward sloping angular lines caused by tension, worry and anxiety are less pleasing. The skin around the eyes is very fine and delicate and it tends to dry out very quickly, which is why lines are easily formed. To counteract this dryness, always use a moisturiser on the area around the eyes. After you have crossed 25 years of age, the application of a little eye cream or special eye oil occasionally will work wonders. Slowly massage with fingers the area around the eyes with oil or cream. Remove surplus cream or oil after about 30 minutes, otherwise your eyes will become puffy.

Pouches under the Eyes

The skin around the eyes is perhaps the most sensitive of all, because the hypo-dermis which exists everywhere else, is absent here. You can never take too much care of your eyes which work all day without much respite. Don't ill treat them. When you are applying cream on them, massage lightly, without exerting pressure. Work from the base of the nose to the temples. Never rub your eyes. Instead of rubbing them, blink your eyelids for the most natural massage. Shut your eyes as tightly as you can, then open them as wide as you can. Repeat this exercise 4 to 5 times, keeping your eyebrows well lifted. Only the eyelids must move. Keep your forehead and face muscles still. This is an excellent exercise for the muscles.

Another exercise is to blink quickly ten times. Shut your eyes, keep them closed for a moment, open them and blink. Rest, blink and rest. Repeat this ten times. This is an excellent exercise for lubricating the eyeballs and toning up the muscles of the eyelids.

Let the eyes have plenty of rest. Giving them rest at night is not enough. During the day, now and again, put the palms of your hands over your eyes and relax. To keep your eyes sparkling, give them plenty of exercise. Roll your eyes around 20 times to the left and 20 times to the right, taking care to close the eyelids when changing directions. Or look at yourself in a mirror, staring straight at the pupils of your eyes, five minutes at each eye. This is a splendid exercise.

Bathe your eyes. To decongest them, there is nothing like an eye lotion, which is readily available in a chemist shop. Bathe your eyes and do not be afraid to keep your eyes wide open. The lotion moistens the mucus, which is temporarily dried up by the constant action of clearing the eyes of thousands of dust particles and other impurities. Don't be afraid to blink while bathing your eyes. Witch-hazel or camomile flower compresses are also excellent for decongesting the eyes. Do not rub the area around the eyes, because rubbing may result in shrinking of the skin. Use the middle finger of the left hand and tap lightly. The skin around the eyes remains healthy by the application of a rose water and cucumber juice mixture. You may use anti-wrinkle cream or hormone cream in case of wrinkles or dark spots around your eyes. Try these home-made remedies:

a) Boil tea leaves and strain. Ferment the area below the eyes with this warm decoction.

b) A light massage by applying almond oil on the skin at night is beneficial. A massage should always be done with outward strokes towards the temples.
c) Wrap oat flour and sandalwood dust in a napkin. Soak it in unheated milk or rose water and rub on the face.

Pock Marks

A pock-marked face is a curse. Make-up can hide these marks but cannot remove them. There are two ways to remove them permanently:

i) *Sand-paper surgery* : This is generally done in foreign countries. It is not prevalent in India due to its exorbitant cost. The drawback is that the patient has to suffer a lot of pain due to numerous small operations on the skin, so these operations should be done by a specialist.

ii) *Skin peeling* : For skin peeling, many kinds of pastes are applied on the patient's face. A layer of the skin gets peeled off after application of every paste and the skin gets spotless after repeating the process many times.

Smallpox spots get reduced with the advancement of age from childhood to adolescence with the growth of the body. Women should look after their skin, specially their face. At night, before sleeping, use deep-cleansing milk and apply a nourishing cream. Facials also reduce these spots. Lanolin cream, which is available in the market, also helps in eliminating them. Soyabean paste fills the deep spots. Apply soyabean paste on the face, let it dry for fifteen to twenty minutes, then wash off with lukewarm water. This process must be repeated thrice a week.

Burns, Scalds and Sunburn

Skin damaged by burning or severe inflammation always leaves scars. Surface injuries often heal with temporary discoloration if the burns are not very severe. The face heals quickly and scars are often unnoticeable. Plastic surgery, if done carefully along the expression lines, makes invisible scars. The backs of the hands heal well, the arms less well and the legs slowly with bad scarring. Bums on the chest and the upper back may produce unpleasant scars which take weeks to heal and also gape open and widen. Minor blemishes or birthmarks should never be removed from these areas for cosmetic reasons as the scar will be worse than the blemish.

Skin Afflictions

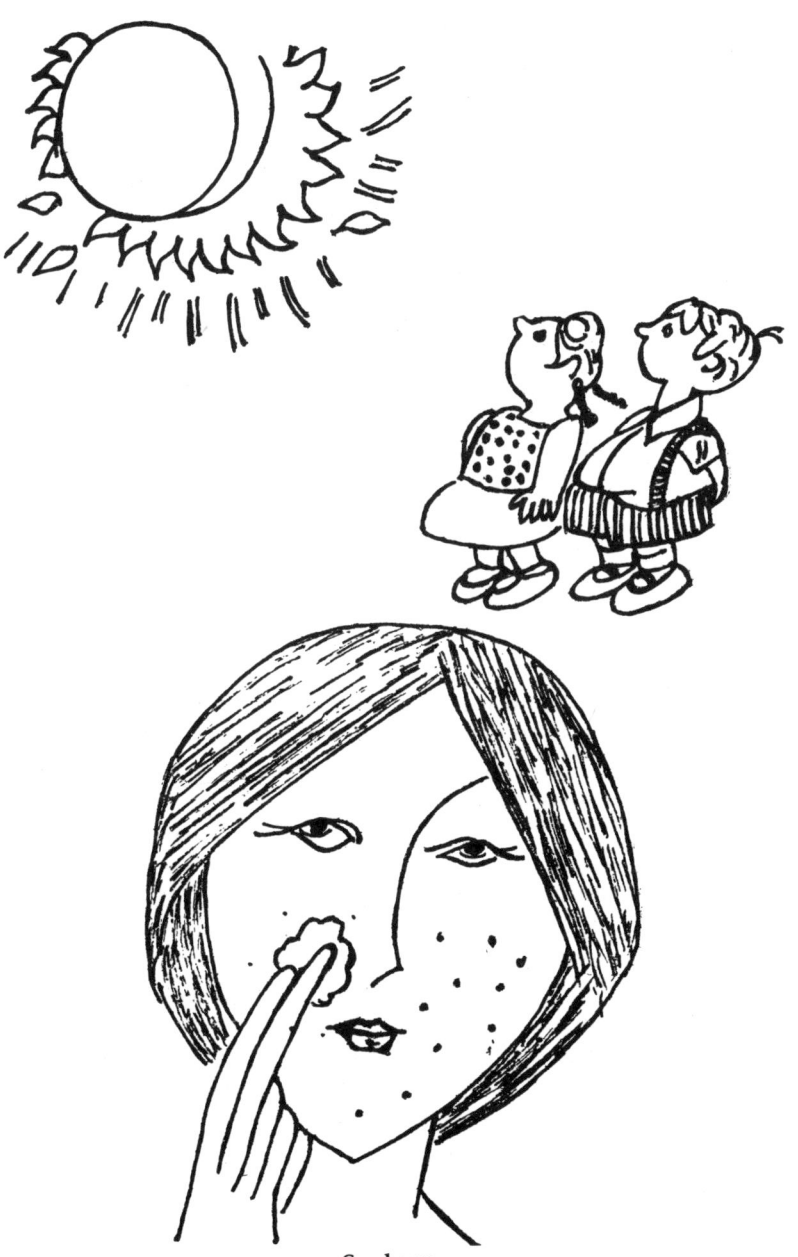

Sunburn

Whereas sunrays are very important for keeping the skin healthy, sunburn is extremely harmful to the skin. As you already know, the sun is a big ball of fire from which many kinds of rays emanate. We can see the rays of light but we cannot see infrared and ultraviolet rays, which are also present. Infrared rays are hot and bring warmth to the body while ultraviolet rays provide Vitamin D to the body which is essential for our health. However the skin gets burnt due to an excess of ultraviolet rays. Melanins, underneath the skin, prevent the skin from getting burnt and that is why blondes or dark-complexioned people get less sunburns than the fair-complexioned people. This is because the darker the skin is, the more the quantity of melanins in the body. The ill-effects of sunrays are maximum on children between six and eight years of age, on women between 25 and 30 years of age and men between 30 and 35 years of age. Ultraviolet rays destroy the melanins in the body and the skin gets darkened. This happens because the minute rays cut the skin and crack it, which results in drying of the skin. The skin then swells and rashes appear on it, after which fresh melanin comes out and the skin gets blackened.

Sunburn reacts on the body in the same way as burning by steam or very hot oil. It results in the drying of skin in swollen blood vessels and damaged cells. Ordinary sunburn can be cured within three or four days but a strong sunburn creates rashes, causing the skin to peel off in layers. Obviously, new cells are born and a new skin does appear again but it is much more drier and thicker than the original one. New skin is often brownish with cracks and it wrinkles easily. These wrinkles are hard to cure. You may benefit from a cold water bath if you are suffering from sunburn, but do not use soap. Remember to protect the skin from the sun until the sunburn gets cured. If rashes appear, consult the specialist. The degree of tolerance of the sun depends upon the nature of the skin. Direct hot sunrays may be more harmful in the month of June when the sun gets nearest to the earth. Sunrays are dangerously hot between 12 noon and 2 o'clock in the afternoon. Drink as much lemon water during this period of the day for a cooling effect.

Sunburn sometimes causes heating of the skin, which is called a burn.

Burns are classified as:

a) *First Degree Burns*
These mild superficial burns cause redness of the skin and later, peeling. For this, no treatment is necessary but calamine lotion is soothing. The burns heal without scarring but there may be temporary darkening or lightening of the skin. Plunging the burnt area in cool water will not lessen the amount of damage but may control the pain to some extent. There are traditional remedies such as applying butter on the affected skin, but these cannot reduce the burn.

b) *Second Degree Burns*
These are more severe, with blistering, swelling and redness of the skin. The blister may be burst with a sterilised needle. The burn should be kept clean and dry, and covered with sterile dressing if necessary. There may be a change in colour for some months, but no permanent scarring.

c) *Third and Fourth Degree Burns*
These cause very serious problems as the whole skin and underlying fat, muscle and tendons are burnt—sometimes down to the bone. The burn is black and charred, but painless, as the nerves are destroyed. Such burns require immediate medical attention because of shock and infection. The complete destruction of the affected skin results in severe scarring when the burn heals.

Sitting too near open fires may cause a mesh of redness and discoloration on the legs which does not fade when away from the heat. This is a chronic low-grade burn and it can also appear on the stomach by hot-water bottles.

Discoloration of Skin

This is often mistaken for scarring. Initially, all scars are red, pink or purple but the colour fades over a year. The blood vessels in a scarred area may be very noticeable but all colour changes can be camouflaged with make-up or a special covering cream. Many scars become temporarily lumpy during healing but later flatten. The skin may darken because of pigments in the skin, the two main pigments deposited in the skin being iron and melanin.

Colour cells (melanocytes) are studded in their millions throughout the skin. They produce a brown pigment called melanin. All races have the same number of colour cells in the skin but they produce different amounts of pigment. In all races the colour production increases by sunshine. The colour of the skin also depends on the blood supply to the skin.

An extensive network of blood vessels runs underneath the epidermis and it reacts to heat and cold. The skin reacts to heat and cold in many ways. Most of the reactions are to the body's advantage, but some are troublesome and a few even dangerous. The body needs a constant internal temperature for all its processes to function properly. The skin regulates body temperature by reducing loss of heat when the weather is cold or prevents extra heat when the body is too hot. We assist the skin in doing this by altering our clothing. Hot weather, warm clothes or a fever causes the body temperature to rise, and sets off the heat-losing mechanisms of the skin, such as reddening of the skin due to enlarging of the blood vessels, swelling of the skin and sweating. The body cools itself by evaporating sweat from the skin. This is the most important way of losing heat. Many skin diseases, especially eczema, provoke the colour cells of the skin to over-produce pigment which drops down into the dermis of the skin and leaves brown marks when the skin trouble disappears. This is called post-inflammatory hyper-pigmentation. Fortunately, the body can slowly remove this pigment and most darkening fades over 1 to 2 years. The darkening is worst in black skin and may occur even after acne. Once this type of colour change has developed, there is little that can remove it except time. The early treatment of the disease will help prevent the colour change.

Increased hormone level in the body during pregnancy stimulates the colour cells of the face and the brown patches appearing specially around the eyes, on the cheeks and on the upper lip. The contraceptive pill can cause similar brown patches. Naturally-occurring hormones cause the problem commonly in women, especially those of Mediterranean origin, who are not on the pill or pregnant, but rarely in men. The brown patches last for many months but usually slowly fade. It is mot important to avoid sunshine which will darken the existing patches. Use sunblocking cream (after consulting your doctor) over the brown patches, together with a sunshade or sun-hat.

Allergies to perfume may produce dark patches on the face and neck. These perfumes may occur in after-shaves, cosmetics and creams in addition to perfume sprays. It is important to wash off all perfumes before sunbathing. Workers exposed to mercury and silver in poor working conditions may get greyish skin on the face and hands. Drugs may cause changes in skin colour which tend to be all over the body and so do some diseases such as liver and glandular diseases and many more. So if you grow brown all over with dark creases of the hand, see your doctor. Very dark patches may develop in later life in the groins and armpits. They can be a sign of illness, so get them checked by a doctor.

Birthmarks

Birthmarks are fairly small moles. However, some birthmarks are very large and brown and more disfiguring. They are often hairy. The only way to deal with this colour change is by surgical removal but this may be very difficult if the birthmark is large, spreads over creases of the body or is of a bizarre shape. Birthmarks are of various types as described below:

Moles (Pigmented nevi)

These are extremely common and harmless lumps in the skin. They are not visible at birth but appear during childhood and early adult life, varying in size and colour from dark brown patches to fleshy bumps. In the early stages, moles may be inflamed and red, but they eventually settle down and become less obvious. If new moles develop after the age of 35, these should be got checked by a doctor. They may become darker and more noticeable during pregnancy, and with the use of contraceptive pills. It is advisable to get a mole removed if:

a) There is an increase in the blackness of the scar.
b) The colour is uneven.
c) There is an increase in the size of a mole.
d) There are changes in the edge of the mole - an uneven or red edge.
e) There are tiny black dots around the mole.
f) There is bleeding or ulcers on the surface of the mole.
g) There are itchy moles.

Port Wine Stains

These are flat red marks usually found on the face and scalp. They cannot be removed by cutting them out. These should be treated by laser as infrared treatment. They can be camouflaged.

Strawberry Marks
This kind of mark is developed soon after a baby is born and grows very rapidly from a bluish small mark to a bluish-red fleshy lump of blood vessels which can bleed. The mark increases in size very fast but eventually shrinks. By the age of ten, only a white scar remains. Avoid surgical treatment as it will cause a worse scar in the end.

Stork's Bill Mark
Some babies have a red birthmark on the nape of the neck which is usually covered by hair.

Dark Patches
Very large areas of brown hairy thinkening may develop on the arms and trunk in the teens. It is not possible to remove them, as large scars are left and these reappear after a short time.

Mangolisan Spots
These occur in babies. They may have bluish birthmarks over the lower back. They are harmless and fade after 18 to 24 months.

Skin Tags
Small tags of skin are very common on the neck and in the armpits and groin. They can be removed by tying fine thread around the stalk. They can also be snipped off with scissors or burnt.

Seborrhoeic Warts
Sometimes, by the age of 60, lots of greasy warts appear on the face, neck and trunk. Very often, people worry about them being evidence of skin cancer. They may become itchy and sore. These can be removed by scraping or freezing.

Skin Cancers
Most skin cancers develop in the very elderly. Too much exposure of fair skins to the sun, past X-ray treatment or exposure to toxic chemicals are some causes. The commonest skin cancer is the Rodent Ulcer. These ulcers usually appear on the face and the skin of the area exposed to the sun. They do not spread elsewhere but grow until removed. "Keratoses" is another form of skin cancer in old age when numerous scaly patches appear on the scalp and other areas, such as the face, ear and backs of the hands. Fleshy rapidly growing lumps or bumps in the skin may spread to the other parts of the body and should be dealt with

immediately. Skin cancer rarely spreads to the rest of the body but needs to be removed by an experienced surgeon by

a) Radiotherapy
b) Surgery or
c) Cryotherapy (liquid nitrogen can be used to kill cancer cells by freezing).

Try to get skin cancer diagnosed at the earliest as it is easier to treat in the early stages. Get it treated by an experienced doctor.

There are several types of skin lightening creams or bleaching creams available in the market which contain a chemical called Hydroquinone which interferes with the production of melanin. These creams cannot lighten the post-inflammatory pigmentation which is the common cause of brown patches though they can lighten the normal skin, birthmarks and freckles. It is generally very irritating to the skin and produces inflammation with more darkening of the skin, or blotchy discoloration. In case of itching and redness, stop using bleaching creams immediately. Use of hydroquinone, especially in high concentration (5% and above) preparations, sometimes damages the underlying tissues, leaving black lumps and cysts. It is better to use 2 per cent hydroquinone, cream unless advised otherwise by a dermatologist. Monobenzyl ether of hydroquinone may contaminate bleaching creams and can cause permanent colour loss which is more disfiguring than the original problem.

Freckles

These are brownish spots on the skin due to precipitation of pigments or exposure to sun. When the skin is sensitive to ultraviolet rays, freckles appear on it. Freckles come in the category of skin disorders but not a skin disease. The following home remedies are useful for this disorder:

1) Grind yellow mustard in milk and apply to the face during the night. Wash you face in the next morning.
2) Mix equal quantities of turmeric and sesame seeds. Grind in water and apply to the face.
3) Take a watermelon, make a hole in its rind and put some grains of rice in it. Take out the rice after a week, grind into a paste and apply on the face.

Boils and Pustules

Boils, the most infective skin condition, are the result of deep bacterial infection of hair follicles. They occur in areas covered with coarse hair which are subjected to repeated mild friction such as the neck, buttocks, knees and elbows. A boil starts as a small, red, painful nodule, increasing in size for a few days, and then becoming soft at its top where the skin gives way to discharge pus. Healing occurs, leaving a tiny scar. A boil usually takes its own course of a week or so in healing and no treatment may be required. But when there are multiple boils, or when a boil becomes large, or when it is on the central portion of the face, systemic antibiotics are required (after consultation with a doctor). If not treated infection can spread to the brain. When the boils tend to occur too frequently, the patient should be investigated for any underlying cause like diabetes, etc.

If the boil is on the nose or the upper lip, the inside of the nose might get inflamed. Boils may sometimes be accompanied by fever. People suffering from boils and pustules should follow the following remedies:

i) Grind neem tree bark in water and apply as a paste.
ii) Grind the bark of the castor tree and the root of biskhapra (*Triathema monogyna*) together and apply as a paste.
iii) Keep your bowels clear and avoid sour or fatty foods.
iv) Eating melons helps the bowels and also cleanses the blood.
v) Take a leaf of the peepal tree, smear it with ghee and apply as a lukewarm bandage on the boil. It will burst in its preliminary stage and the growth will subside.

Prickly Heat

This is a very common condition during hot days and occurs during the hot summer and rainy season when there is profuse sweating and the body is not exposed to the air. Red pustules of the size of mustard grains appear on the body, especially on the chest, back and the abdomen. There is intense itching and if the affected skin area is scratched, it gives temporary relief, though there are chances of the skin getting septic. Persons subjected to prickly heat should avoid heavy garments and try to expose the affected area to air. Cold water baths twice every day will helps as will the following easy remedies too :

1) Dissolve Fuller's earth *(Multani Mitti)* in water to make a thin paste. It should be smeared over the affected parts. When the paste has dried, wash it with cold water.
2) Apply green henna, ground in water, on the affected skin.

3) Grind leaves of neem in water and apply on the affected skin.
4) The most effective remedy for treating prickly heat is to take a small piece of sandalwood and rub it on a stone with rose water. Mix a pinch of powdered alum and apply to the affected skin twice or thrice a week, depending upon the condition of prickly heat.
5) Another way to treat prickly heat is to dissolve a tablespoon of sada bicarbonate in half a cup of water and mix in one tablespoon of rose water. Apply it to the affected skin with cotton wool.

Red Nose

Diet plays an important part in this condition. A red nose is very common with hearty eaters and heavy drinkers but the trouble may arise from a delicate skin too. If so, avoid sudden changes of temperature. Here is an excellent and effective home remedy:

Take rose water lotion or put a little tannin in some glycerine, and massage your nose up and down, taking care to use only two fingers. Hold your nose between two fingers.

Whitlow: The Chronic Paronychia

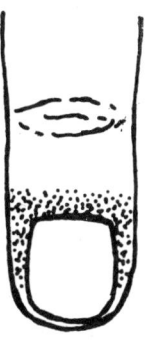

Whitlow is a term applied to all acute inflammations of the deep-seated tissues in the finger, whether the structure is affected by the root of the nail, the pulp of the fingertips, the skin of fingers or the bone. In this condition, a small painful abscess forms at the base of the nail or the pulp of the finger. Sometimes, the patient feels intense pain as the bursting of an abscess takes a long time. Frequently occurring in housewives, chronic paronychia is an infection of the nail fold with a yeast-like fungus called candida. The predisposing factor is the prolonged wetting of hands. The condition usually starts in one finger (generally, the middle finger of the right hand) as a glazed red swelling of the nail fold. Later, other fingers may be affected. Secondary infection with bacteria causes pain and discharge of pus from the nail fold. Sometimes the nail is lost and the finger may be disfigured. It is essential to keep hands dry as far as possible to make healing possible quickly. Local application of 1 per cent Gention—violet paint of mycostatin suspension (P)—in the nail fold twice everyday for a prolonged period would help cure the disease. Here is a home remedy : Mix one part of isphagula in four parts of vinegar, and apply to the infected spot. The poultice - like mixture should be bandaged with clean cloth and water sprinkled over it. The bandage should be changed after every 3 to 4 hours. The inflammation will subside in 2 to 3 days. Once the pus has been ejected, cooked leaves of neem should be wrapped over the site of the whitlow.

Chilblains and Cracked Skin
Chilblains, an abnormal reaction to cold which occurs in some individuals, develop with the onset of winter. Young people, especially girls, are more often affected. That is the reason why, particularly during winter, the lips can get chapped and the skin of the hands crack because of defective functioning of the sebaceous glands. Chilblains consist of a bluish-red discoloration, swelling and sometimes blistering of toes and/or fingers. Very rarely, the nose, ears and cheeks may be involved. The affected person experiences severe itching or burning. The condition heals with the arrival of summer but may recur every winter.

As a therapeutic and prophylactic measure, the patient should keep himself warm with the use of properly fitting gloves and socks. Peripheral vasodilators like Nicotinic Acid and Isoxuprin (also known as Duvadilan) can give relief to symptoms in more than 50 per cent of the cases. Ulcers produced from ruptured blisters should be properly dressed with antibiotic creams. There are several easy home remedies for cracked skin. The hands should be properly scrubbed, dried and then smeared with ghee or mustard oil. The best application is the cream that forms over boiled milk when it has cooled down. It should be applied and massaged during night just before going to bed. Even chapped lips can be smeared with this cream at night. On waking up, you will find the lips tender and soft as they should be.

Red Veins on Cheeks
These usually indicate a sensitive skin that has been neglected or ill-treated. The skin is very thin and the blood vessels are very near the surface. They are affected readily by poor circulation or

by extremes of temperature and washing the face with very hot water or splashing it with icy cold water usually causes this condition and sometimes makes it much worse. If you suffer from broken veins, protect the skin from weather conditions by using a moisturiser. But special lotions and waxy creams should be used in high altitudes to give the skin added protection. Avoid going from one extreme of temperature to another and always wait a few minutes in between in a place with intermediate temperature. Avoid rich, spicy foods, hot drinks and alcohol when you suffer from this condition. It is also possible to have treatment with an electrical process which drains the blocked blood vessels and seals them. This process is not common in India. Moisturisers are very useful for this skin disorder.

Moisturisers, band creams, body lotions, etc., all work on the same principle. The skin looks its best when it contains the maximum amount of water. Moisturisers do this either by applying a water-holding substance (humectant) such as urea or polyethylene glycol or by using an oil or grease to prevent water from evaporating from the skin. The greasy water-in-oil emulsions are more satisfactory than lighter oil-in-water ones. These are best applied to skin with a high water content, after bathing, washing or steaming the face. The choice of moisturisers depends on one's skin. For face, eyes, lips, neck, hands and body, a single moisturiser is enough but night creams are greasier than day creams. Most moisturisers also make the skin feel smoother by lubricating it with oil, and make it look smoother by sticking down the fine scales. Here's an easy to make home-made moisturising cream:

Collect the following ingredients:
2 tablespoons beeswax
1 tablespoon liquid wax
5 teaspoons almond oil
4 teaspoons water
a few drops of scented oil or scent

Process : Melt the beeswax and liquid wax in a china bowl. Add almond oil to it. Heat water in another container and then mix it in the first mixture. Remember that both mixtures should be prepared at the same temperatures. Stir the thick mixture with a wooden spoon till it gets cold. During the cooling process, add scent to it.

Hypersensitive Skin

These are very delicate skins and need a lot of care and attention. They may be the types which are allergic to various kinds of cosmetics such as creams, powders and perfumes. They may react violently when there is a change in temperature, becoming red, blotchy and broken-veined. The important thing is to find out what your skin likes and dislikes. If any cosmetic causes swelling or irritation, switch to another make or try some special non-allergic cosmetics suitable for hypersensitive skins. These are available with leading chemists or large stores. Never wash such skins with too hot or very cold water. Avoid the use of soap as far as possible.

Blotchiness

Dry skin is more sensitive than a moist one. People who have skin liable to be blotchy must avoid exposing it to excessive heat or excessive cold, since rapid changes of temperature always have harmful effects on skins. Avoid the use of soap as it is harmful for blotchy skins. Instead, use cow's unboiled milk or a cleansing milk with a lanolin base. Do not use a spirit tonic lotion. Here are few useful tips for blotchy skins:

a) Cover your skin when going out with a good cream, which can be either purchased from the market of which you may prepare yourself. Collect the following ingredients:

- 2 teaspoons beeswax
- 2 teaspoons emulsifying wax
- 8 teaspoons almond oil
- 4 teaspoons lanolin
- 4 teaspoons coconut oil
- 6 teaspoons orange flower water
- 3 drops tincture benzoin

Process : Melt the beeswax, emulsifying wax, almond oil, lanolin and coconut oil on medium heat and simultaneously stir it. Now add orange flower water gradually, but keep on stirring. When the mixture becomes thick, remove it from the heat. Cool and fill in a bottle.

b) Use body lotion on the skin of your body an hour before you go for a bath. Here is home-made recipe for this:

Collect the following ingredients:
- 1/2 tablespoon lanolin
- 1 tablespoon petroleum jelly

4 tablespoons mineral oil
8 teaspoons clean water
1 tablespoon rose water
5 drops violet extract

Process : Melt lanolin, petroleum jelly and mineral oil on medium heat. Heat clean water and violet extract in another bowl and mix the contents of the two containers and stir till it cools down.

Cold Sores

Cold sores occur most commonly on the lips, though they can develop on any part of the body. They are a result of a virus: Herpes simplex. This virus sometimes also affects the genitalia of adults. This type of infection is spread by sexual intercourse and forms one of the many sexually-transmitted diseases. The virus of cold sores generally lies dormant in the body, but can be activated by colds, fevers, stressful conditions, emotional upheavals or any serious illness. It is best to avoid intimate contact with an individual who is having an attack of herpes. For an acute attack, here are a couple of remedies:

a) Cold compresses or ice can relieve the pain.
b) Ether compresses would hasten healing.
c) Acyclovir, a new treatment for herpes, can give considerable relief to persons getting recurrent attacks.

(The above treatment should be given only after consultation with a doctor)

Face Lifting and Peeling

Lifting — the name of this operation — describes the procedure itself in that the very skin is lifted. Wrinkled skin can be cured by this method. The surgeon makes an incision at the level of the temples, lifts the skin from the cheeks and draws it upwards. The rejuvenating effect is amazing, but it is by no means a permanent cure. Lifting may last some years, after which it has to be done again.

If the skin is pitted with scars left by pimples, or has strawberry marks and minor scars, or has lost its radiance and continues to look muddy, in spite of the care you are giving it, consult a dermatologist for "peeling treatment". Peeling means the simple deep-cleansing accomplished by removing a very thin layer of skin. Of course, this operation must be very delicately performed by a skin specialist. If these marks cannot be removed by the peeling treatment, skin surgery can reduce them to such an extent that they will be almost unnoticeable. Minor scars can be dealt with by electric treatment, by rubbing carbon snow, by ultraviolet rays treatment and by cortisone injections; very disfiguring scars can be made less noticeable by grafting and lifting as discussed above.

Relaxation, washing and beauty care which suit our type of skin are your best weapons against wrinkles. For some men and women, wrinkles represent the end of the struggle. For others it is an alarming signal to rush to the skin specialists. Here again you cannot expect miracles. Self-discipline and daily beauty care are the best preventives. It is fortunate that we have at our disposal efficient, simple and inexpensive remedies such as self-massage and masks. Here is an anti-wrinkle home preparation cream:

Collect a teaspoonful of honey, a few drops of lemon juice and a drop of sweet almond oil. Mix together and apply on your face, keeping your eyes shut. Let it dry for 20 minutes, then wash.

3

SKIN DISEASES

Treatment of Pimples

Skin complaints mar many a lovely skin. The scars left by pimples and acne are usually the result of negligence. Pimples are a serious problem at the adolescent stage. They appear on the cheeks, forehead and nose and spoil the appearance. Eight out of ten teenagers suffer from this problem but though it cannot be prevented or cured at present, proper treatment will control or minimise it to some extent.

Why do pimples appear in youth? The answer to this question is that as soon as one crosses childhood and enters the threshold of adolescence, different parts of the body start developing. The oil-glands underneath the skin become overactive and ooze grease which blocks the skin pores, causing pimples to sprout.

I would suggest the following home remedies :
a) Use sulpher soap to keep the oil-glands clean.
b) Remove make-up at night before going to bed.
c) Steam your face once a week to keep the pores open.
d) A *Multani Mitti* pack is an effective way to control pimples.
e) Take a spoonful of honey mixed with rose water daily.
f) Apply cucumber juice mixed with rose water.
g) Cut down blood-heating foods, such as sweets, fats and spicy dishes.
h) Do not squeeze pimples—the skin may become septic and leave behind permanent marks which damage your looks.
i) Do not neglect pimples.

Methods and medication for treating acne vary from one doctor to another and its treatment also varies with the needs of the individual patient. After trying self-treatment and finding no success, consult your doctor. The treatment often involves nothing more than simple local skin care. Control of acne is a long term, continuing process. Follow the instructions of your doctor faithfully and regularly.

Acne and Its Cure

Acne is very common in the teens and twenties. Sometimes acne is not caused by germs or dirt. The male sex hormones (androgens) cause acne. When boys attain puberty the androgens cause the voice to break, a beard to grow, the skin to become greasy and spots to erupt. All women have both female hormones (oestrogen and progesterone) and androgens. Acne is due to an imbalance of these hormones and not due to extra male hormones. Greasy skin, excess facial and body hair, and the thinning of scalp hair can also be due to this imbalance. Most people grow out of acne in their twenties, some as late as the thirties.

In most women, changes in the balance of female hormones during menstruation cause a few acne spots each month. Oral contraceptive pills may either improve acne or make it worse. The chin area is often the worse affected in older women and the shoulders, back and chest are affected worse than the face. Blackheads, spots and lumps of acne are all related to the sebaleous glands which produce grease (known as sebum).

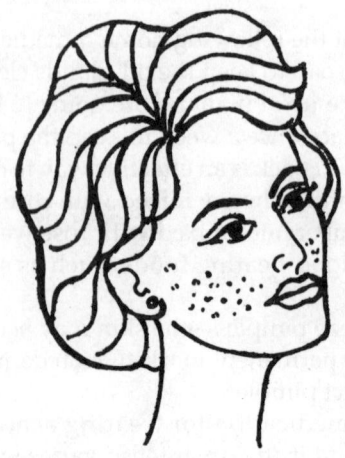

Acne scars

Androgen increases the amount of grease formed and blocks the opening of the glands. The blockage is visible as a blackhead and the glands become swollen and inflamed.

Bad acne needs a doctor's help before you get depressed and discouraged. Acne preparations will not cure bad acne. There is a vast and bewildering array of preparations for acne—lotions, gels, creams, ointments, scrubs and soaps. Many are slightly beneficial while some are harmful.

Peeling of the skin opens up the pores and helps in removing blackheads and small spots. Face masks, abrasive scrubs, and sponges also unblock the pores. Most acne preparations are peeling agents which contain benzoyl peroxide. Preparations containing other ingredients such as rescorcinol sulphur, or antiseptics are not as good. So check the ingredients before you buy peeling agents. Brasivol and Ionax are common peeling agents available in the market.

Antibiotic lotions containing Clindamycin or Erythromycin are successful in treating acne, but consult a doctor before using such lotions. Other antibiotic lotions are not so useful.

Retinoic acid (from Vitamin A) slowly clears blackheads if applied on the skin but the disadvantages are peeling, drying, and darkening of skin.

Antibiotics are very effective as they suppress the inflammation of acne spots and cut down skin bacteria. Tetracyclines, Erythromycin and Septrin are most commonly used. Antibiotics are taken in very long courses, usually nine months or more. The acne clears in 2 to 6 months, after which the quality of the dosage is slowly reduced every three months or so. Many people need one tablet a day or less for years to keep the skin clear. There are no long-term side effects from this but the treatment should be taken with the consultation of a qualified skin specialist.

The following home remedies should be tried for acne:
1) Mix slake lime in water (one part lime should be mixed with 20 parts water) and mix with finely powdered sulphur (2 parts). Boil the mixture till half the quantity is left. Apply a light coat of the fluid to the acne areas.
2) Grind the bark of neem and turmeric (*haldi*) together in water. Ruf the paste on the affected parts.

3) Rub a piece of sandalwood on a clean stone, using a little of rose water or cucumber juice to make a paste. This pack will give you a tingling, fresh feeling and will discourage pimples and acne.

Home Facials for Acne Skin

Acne is common in teens and twenties, and is a serious disorder of the sebaceous glands, requiring medical direction. To keep skin conditions under control, observe the following suggestions:
 a) Reduce the oiliness of the skin.
 b) Remove the blackheads.
 c) Regularly cleanse the skin.
 d) Use special medicated preparations.
 e) Have a well-balanced, regular diet.

Home facials for acne skin should followed thus:
1) Cleanse the face with medicated soap and warm water.
2) Apply acne cream or ointment all over the face and the neck.
3) Apply high frequency current over the affected skin for not more than five minutes. Then remove the acne cream with tissues.
4) Apply a suitable face mask and keep it on for ten minutes.
5) Remove the mask and blot the residue with a cold, wet towel.
6) Saturate cotton with an astringent lotion and apply with a blotting movement.
7) Moisten a piece of cotton with an antiseptic lotion and touch each and every pimple or acne.
8) Never apply make-up on an acne skin.

All teenagers have some acne, varying from a few blackheads to a very unsightly and upsetting problem of large pus-filled spots. Steaming is an excellent way to clean all types of skin. It cleans the skin, stimulates the circulation and unclogs the blocked pores. Electrical devices are available to produce steam—this process is known as a sauna facial.

If your skin is dry, steam your face once a week. In the case of oily skins, steaming can be done daily.

Steaming should be done by leaning over a large bowl of boiling water. Cover your head with a towel, making a tent around the bowl. Do not get too close to the boiling water, for if the steam is too hot, it might cause broken veins.

Skin Diseases

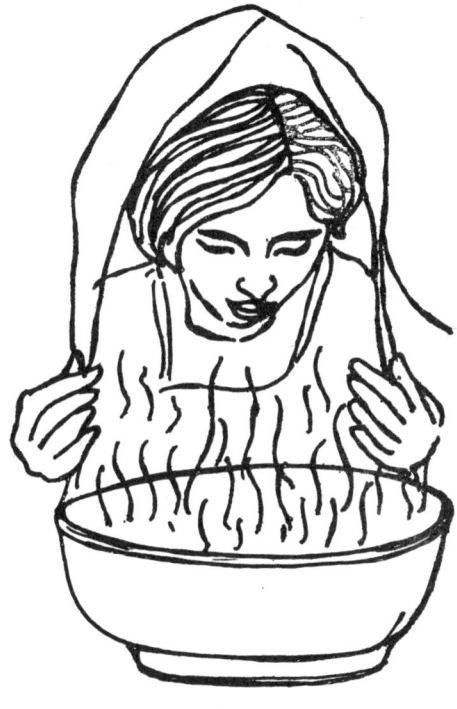

Steaming

Antibiotic lotions are also successful in treating acne but it takes about two months to work and your doctor's advice is a must.

Warts on the Face

The concept of beauty in the general sense is based on a smooth, silky skin with a smooth texture and colour. Blemishes of any kind, sometimes in the form of nevi or warts, are considered ugly. Though some may consider them as "Beauty spots", in general, they are not really welcome.

Warts are small epidermic growths caused by a virus. These growths vary in size and shape and are commonly of three types: Plane warts, Common warts and Planter warts.

Plane warts are the simplest of all warts. They are usually small, smooth and skin-coloured or brownish lesions which are raised slightly from the skin surface. They usually occur in the face and outer surface of the hands. The most commonly affected are children and young adults.

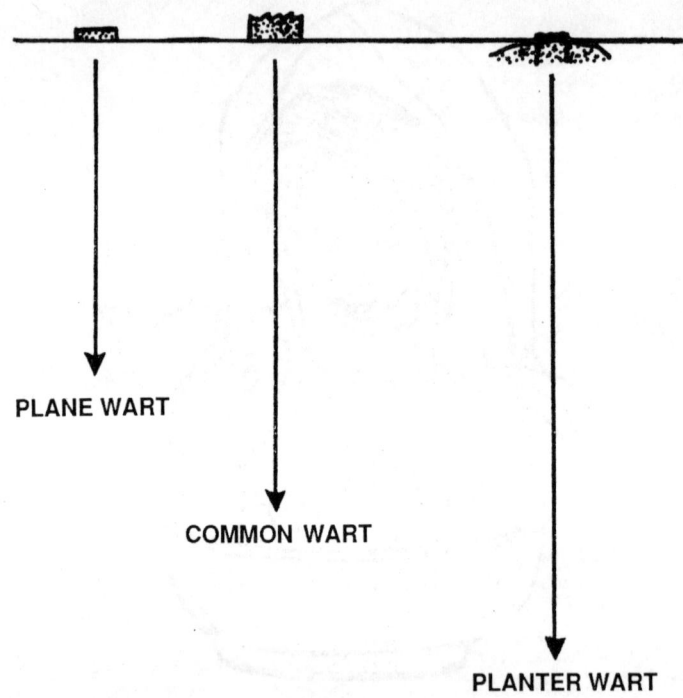

Cross-section of different types of warts

Common warts are larger and firmer elevations with a rough surface. They usually occur on the hands, forearms, knees and the upper parts of the feet. People usually develop thickening of the skin surface at the weight-bearing area in the sole (planter surface of the feet). Commonly known as corns they are caused by consistent pressure at a particular area which makes the outermost, horny layer of the skin proliferate. Planter warts are slightly different. They normally contain blood vessels and the surface of the wart, if carefully pared, bleeds because of this.

Pain is characteristic of both corns and warts. If you press a corn vertically on the top with a blunt object, it is markedly tender; whereas in planter warts tenderness is felt when pressed from the sides.

A mole or a nevus is synonymous with a birthmark. It is a discoloration of a circumscribed area of the skin due to extra pigment deposition. A mole is darker in colour and is solid. In comparison, a wart is a softer structure which is translucent and marked with veins.

Warts and nevi are blemishes and mar the face. Besides the cosmetic aspect, planter warts, being painful, do not permit the sufferer to walk properly, the weight-bearing areas are painful and cannot take any pressure, resulting in uneven weight distribution to other areas of the feet which are not supposed to transmit the body weight. The result is obvious. The gait of a person becomes faulty and his feet arches are strained. This further leads to malalignments of the joints and eventually may become one of the causes of arthritis.

While seeking treatment for warts, it is important to remember that warts can disappear spontaneously. This is specially true of plane warts in children where the therapy is not only disappointing but may result in scars. It is, therefore, worthwhile waiting for a few years before considering actual treatment of warts in the case of children. The treatment of warts consists in eliminating them either by chemical lotion or physical means. A peeling agent like 4 per cent sulphur calamine lotion or Retino A cream applied daily, may be all that is needed to remove plane warts.

Common warts are best treated by electro-cautery. Under local anaesthesia, the warts are removed with a cautery which excises the wart with an electric current while cauterising the site. Alternatively, they can also be scooped out with a curette under local anaesthesia, by cauterising the site with electro-cautery.

Freezing the wart with liquid nitrogen or carbon-snow is another effective method. Planter warts can also be treated by curettage combined with electro-cautery. More conservative methods like application of Salicylic acid in paste form under occlusion daily for two to three weeks may also cure warts.

Warts are simple afflictions, not a threat to life, but they can be quite troublesome and may cripple the smooth running of day to day life, if one is overconscious of them. While there is a slight danger of complications developing in these extra growths of skin, by and large, they are amenable to simple cures.

Genital warts are transmitted by contact in the sexually active. They may be related to the development of cervical cancer. So if you have warts, get them treated properly and have regular cervical smears. Salicylic acid plasters, Salicylic acid collodion, Salactol and Duofilm are common wart preparations available.

Contagious Diseases of the Skin : Scabies

Scabies is a contagious disease caused by a mite - Sorcoptes scabies. The usual mode of infection is by direct contact between bedfellows, or children who hold hands while playing. Though infected bedclothes and undergarments could spread the disease, it seems to be a rather uncommon mode.

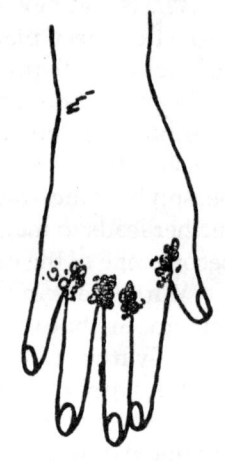

The most prominent symptom of scabies is itching, which is often most severe at night. The lesions are most pronounced on webs between the fingers, wrists, elbows, around the armpits, abdomen, buttocks and the inner sides of the thighs. Very often external genitalia in males and breasts in females are also affected. The face, however, is always spared except in infants. The most important lesion which is almost diagnostic is a burrow. It appears as a whitish or a black zig zag line of about 6-12 mm length, caused by the mite burrowing horizontally in the horny layer of the epidermis. In addition, there are inflammatory papules and some vesicles. Scratching might result in the lesions getting secondarily infected with bacteria-producing pus containing lesions of impetigo, boils, abscesses, etc. It is to be remembered that scabies is no respecter of persons. And a person of high social standing, with a good record of personal hygiene is not immune to contracting this disease. In such instances, it is likely that the clinical picture of a rash may not be typical and there may be only a few lesions.

How to Treat Scabies

Scabies is treated with the local application of 25 per cent benzyl benzoate emulsion (Ascabiol) or 10 per cent gammabenzene hexachloride (Scabiezima, Scarab). It is important that all the members of the family are simultaneously treated. Before using the medicine, the patient must have a thorough scrubbing, and a bath with soap and water. The lotion is applied all over the body except on the face. The applications are repeated at twelve-hourly intervals and a total of 3 to 4 applications are sufficient. After 48 hours of the first application, the patient should again have a bath. It is important that either the hands are not washed at all during these 48 hours or if washed, a second coating of the application is done immediately afterwards. The clothes must be changed at the end of the treatment and laundered. (Scabies should be treated with the consultation of a doctor only.)

Thrush (Candida)
Thrush is another common infection which can cause sores at the angles of the mouth, especially in denture wearers where it lurks above the dental plate. Babies may get white patches of thrush on the tongue and on the sides of the mouth. Thrush infection of vagina with itching and discharge is also common and many women have thrush in several places at once. Vaginal thrush usually clears with pessaries such as Nystatin and Clotrimazole. Contraceptive pills, antibiotics and pregnancy can create conditions which encourage thrush. Avoid nylon panties, tight jeans and a moist environment. Hands frequently immersed in water or cuticles pushed back can suffer redness and swelling around the fingernails due to thrush infection. To help stop nail problems, avoid water by wearing rubber or plastic gloves. For mouth problems, wear better fitting false teeth, take them out at night and scrub the dentures well with a nail-brush.

Skin Inflammations
There are several types of skin inflammations, such as Dermatitis, Eczema, Psoriasis, Herpes simplex and skin disorders due to the use of cosmetics. Some of these are described below:

1) *Dermatitis*
Dermatitis is the term used to signify an inflammatory condition of the skin. The skin lesions appear in various forms, such as vesicles or papules.

2) *Eczema*
Eczema is an inflammation of the skin of an acute or chronic nature. It is frequently accompanied by itching and various other unpleasant sensations. It should be referred to a physician or a skin specialist for treatment.

3) *Psoriasis*

Psoriasis is a common, chronic, inflammatory skin disease, the cause of which is unknown. It is usually found on the scalp, elbows, knees, chest and the lower back. It rarely affects the face, and can be spread by irritation.

4) *Herpes Simplex and Herpes Zoster*

Herpes simplex is a virus infection of unknown origin, and is commonly known as "Blisters". The blisters usually appear on the lips, nostrils or any part of the face. Herpes zoster is caused by the same virus as chickenpox. Genital herpes is another virus which causes chickenpox. Common in young people, this is caused by a different strain of the same virus, caught by having sex with someone who has herpes. Groups of little blisters appear on the genital area, thighs and buttocks. They are painful, tender and highly infectious. The first infection is the worst, with swollen glands and temperature. The blisters crust over and clear in about a week's time. The virus becomes dormant but may cause repeated attacks.

5) *Skin Allergies*

Skin disorders due to the use of cosmetics are generally called skin allergies. Some individuals may develop allergies due to certain cosmetic preparations containing chemicals, which include cold wave lotions, hair sprays, tints, lipsticks and cosmetics for eye make-up.

Allergies are fashionable and many people assume their skin trouble is due to an allergy but this is rarely true. In fact, hardly 5 per cent of all patients attending skin clinics are suffering from a true allergy. An allergic rash can be caused by a substance coming into contact with the skin which is known as "Contact Allergy". Or an allergy can be a reaction to some substance entering the body. There are two kinds of contact allergy : eczema and nettle rash (also known as contact urticaria). Contact eczema (contact dermatitis) is the commonest type of allergy. The skin reacts to contact with a substance called allergen by becoming red and itchy. In a very severe reaction, the skin blisters or 'weeps'. Swelling may be caused and usually affects the eyes, if the face is affected. The rash persists for weeks or months. The contact allergy is of many types which shall be discussed in detail in this chapter. Contact urticaria is a rare kind of allergy and usually people react within minutes with weals due to skin contact with certain foods and substances taken internally.

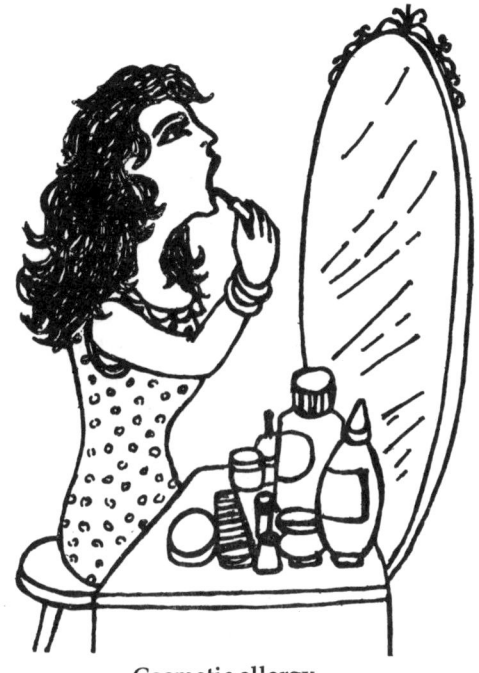

Cosmetic allergy

Urticaria

Hives is a temporary swelling of the skin, caused by a localised collection of fluid in the dermis due to leakage from blood vessels. It can result from any of the following:
 a) Allergy to foods, pollens and drugs.
 b) Change in the temperature.
 c) Infections, including the presence of worms.
 d) Emotional upsets.

Sometimes, the cause cannot be accurately determined but if the cause can be made out, it is easy to cure urticaria. If the cause is not obvious, then a very effective way to get relief is to use anti-allergic drugs for some weeks (with the consultancy of your doctor) till the problem subsides.

Urticaria is an eruption of weals. Weals, the itching, pale or pink, edematous, raised lesions resembling those caused by the sting of a nettle, last for a short time of a few hours only, but reappear at the same or different sites. On areas like lips, eyelids and groins, edematous swellings may erupt because of the looseness of subcutaneous tissue where a large amount of fluid can accumulate. Urticaria is a reaction pattern of the skin which can be caused by a number of factors. The common ones are:

1. Allergic urticaria is the commonest allergic condition of the skin. Substances which cause allergic urticaria enter the body by inhalation or injections. Drugs like penicillin, sulphonamides, aspirin, tetracyclines and even B complex vitamins are among the commonest causes of urticaria. Aspirin can also cause urticaria by non-allergic means. Many foods like fish, pork, eggs, mushroom, milk, wheat, rice and pulses, etc., can also cause urticaria. Pollens, dust, horse dander, etc., can be inhaled and cause urticaria, though more frequently they are a cause of naso-respiratory allergy. Vaccines and anti-toxin injections can also cause urticaria. Some parasitic infections of the intestines and the stings of mosquitoes, wasps and bees can also cause widespread allergic urticaria. At times a focus of infection in the throat, sinuses, ears, teeth or kidney may be the cause of urticaria.

2. Physical factors like cold, heat, exertion, ultraviolet radiation and pressure can produce urticaria in sensitive individuals.

3. Psychological stress resulting from sex problems and problems regarding employment, family and finances have been known to cause urticaria in some persons.

In all cases of urticaria, a careful history is taken, especially with regard to drug intake, relationship of urticaria with ingestion of any particular food or any of the physical factors mentioned above. A psychological assessment of the patient is also made. A physical examination is important to exclude or confirm the presence of a focus of infection or some other underlying disease. Microscopic stool examination is done to detect any intestinal worm infestation. The prick and intra-dermal tests on the skin, used for identification of allergy in asthma, are generally unless in urticaria.

Suppressive treatment of urticaria is carried out by administering antihistaminic drugs like Chloropheneramine (Avil) triprolidine hydrochloride, Actidil and Cyproheptadine hydrochloride (Periactin). The dose and the frequency should be adjusted to give adequate coverage for 24 hours. All these drugs cause varying degrees of drowsiness, hence driving, operating machines and other jobs which require mental alertness should be avoided while undergoing treatment. Urticaria, if not responsive to oral antihistamines, may have to be treated with injections of adrenaline or steroids especially for patients complaining of a choking sensation in the throat which occurs due to swelling in the respiratory passage.

Psoriasis
It is a common, chronic, inflammatory skin disease, the cause of which is unknown. It is usually found on the scalp, elbows, knees, chest and the lower back. It is rarely on the face, and can be spread by irritation. Psoriasis is a very common disease in Britain; it is estimated that 1-2 million people suffer from it. The main problem is that the skin grows too rapidly in some places, forming a silvery scale over thick patches which become inflamed and red. Patches of psoriasis develop over areas where the skin is frequently knocked or has been injured in grazes, cuts and operation scars. The scalp is badly affected and the scaling gives rise to hard lumps and very flaky dandruff. Psoriasis is harmless but can become very distressing as it can be very difficult to cope mentally with the appearance of the skin. Many sufferers dislike exposing their skin when sunbathing or playing sports. Moreover, painful fissures can be troublesome and itching can be a nuisance.

This chronic disease of the skin manifests itself in patches of redness accompanied by loose silvery white scales. It has been observed that one-fourth of psoriasis patients, have other family members who also suffer from the same disease, indicating that psoriasis is hereditary. The condition can start at any age. The number and extent of lesions differs from patient to patient and in a given patient from time to time. There may be only a few lesions or the whole body may be involved. Most people start to get patches between the ages of 15 and 25, but it can develop at any age from childhood to extreme old age. I have seen a person who was 95 when he first developed the problem. The attacks of psoriasis may be triggered by an illness, especially a sore throat, an operation, the use of certain drugs, an injury or sunburn.

Psoriasis tends to get better in summer and worse in winter but tends to come and go on its own and may clear up completely for years before a new patch develops. As stated earlier, the very common sites of involvement are usually the scalp, elbows, knees and buttocks. Scalp lesions are well defined and are covered with a rather heavy mass of scales as opposed to seborrhoeic dermatitis, where there is a diffused involvement of the whole scalp and the scaling is not so heavy. Nails, in more than 50 per cent of the psoriatics, show some abnormality like pitting, ridging or thickening and discoloration. One to two per cent of psoriatic patients may develop pain in the joints, especially in the distal joints on fingers. An overweight individual with psoriasis should resort to systematic weight reduction. Patients who are not overweight are best advised to eat as balanced a diet as possible. The aim of treatment in psoriasis is to bring about a remission as early as possible and to maintain it for as long a period as possible.

Most psoriasis treatments are ointments based on coal tar and dithranol. Consult your doctor before starting a treatment. These ointments can be very effective although they take some time (sometimes many months to work). They are smelly and stain clothes and the skin, so it is best to apply them at night when going to sleep and to use old sheets. Dithranol can burn the eteroids like 1 per cent Hydrocortisone or Betamethasone velerate 0.1 per cent are used for treatment. In patients with limited involvement, Corticosteroids can also be applied under occlusion. A recent mode of treatment in vogue in the United States is to administer Methoxy psorlen (a sun sensitiser) and expose the body to ultraviolet light. For this purpose specially constructed chambers lined with ultraviolet lamps are available. The long-term effects of this method are yet to be fully assessed and the theoretical risk of cancer developing by this method is already worrying some researchers.

Ultraviolet radiation from sunshine, for example, 2 to 3 weeks of sunbathing, may clear your psoriasis for some months. Ultraviolet lamps will also help and may be helpful in 4 to 6 weeks courses but should be used longer only on your doctor's advice as prolonged treatment may have harmful long-term effects. Sunburn must be avoided as this will worsen the psoriasis. Sunbeds and ultraviolet A (UVA) lamps will really improve the psoriasis if used in combination with drugs called Psoralens (PUVA). Regular PUVA treatment will usually control

Skin Diseases

bad psoriasis, but increase the risk of skin ageing and skin cancer, especially in fair skin. The treatment is used only for bad psoriasis and under medical supervision.

Many of the anticancer drugs will slow down skin growth and control psoriasis. However, they usually have unpleasant side effects. Methotrexate is used in very severe psoriasis and has to be taken continuously. Regular liver and blood checks are essential. New drugs derived from Vitamin A (Retinoids) have been used for psoriasis but they also cause liver and blood problems and are used only in severe cases.

Leucoderma : The Whitening of Skin

To have white spots or patches on the body is a disease. Due to loss of pigmentation in the skin, white patches of varying sizes and shapes make their appearance on the body. This disease is called leucoderma. The white patches on the skin are painless but a leucoderma patient is more embarrassed than a victim of any pain or discomfort as in addition to being a medical and beauty problem, it also becomes a social stigma. Leucoderma is curable and is not a contagious disease. An imbalance of melanin in the body results in the appearance of white spots. These white patches are a curse for women and are directly related to the nature of the skin. Darker skins have more patches because such skins contain more melanins. It must be clarified here that white patches are not congenital nor hereditary. Children are not affected if the mother has these patches. It is also erroneous to think that a woman who has leucoderma does not enjoy marital pleasures.

Often, people believe that the condition is caused by eating fish or mutton along with milk. But it is not so, because even vegetarians are prone to it. Detection of the disease in the first six months makes it easier to cure. But if it is left untreated, it may become intractable. The seeds of Babchi are useful in treating leucoderma. The seeds are steeped in ginger juice for 72 hours and then rubbed with the hands to remove the husk, dried and powdered. The ground seeds should be applied to the white spots. Another useful application is the juice of the leaves of Goose Foot (*Bathua*). It should be applied to the white spots three to four times a day. A "Chandan" pack is very useful in treating leucoderma. The leucoderma patient must be kept on a salt-free diet but rock salt may be permitted in minute quantities. The white spots should be also protected from exposure to heat.

In fact, family history is present in only six to eight per cent of patients with leucoderma. The remaining 92 to 94 per cent of patients have never had a patient with the disease in the family for the last three to four generations. Many patients develop the disease rather suddenly for no obvious reason. It is indeed difficult to make an exact forecast for this disease.

Leprosy
The symptoms of this disease are that the skin starts whitening, round lumps are formed, fingers starts crumbling and eyesight is affected. A doctor should immediately be consulted. The disease can be hereditary and it is perhaps the most serious and also the most disgusting disorder of the skin. The disease is endemic to tropical climates. If treatment is not given in the initial stage, it will damage the skin. Leprosy is infectious also and affects not only the skin but also the nerves. Leprosy is of two types : Tuberculoid and Lepromatous.

Tuberculoid leprosy is not very serious and is self-healing. The symptoms found in both types of leprosy are similar, and one cannot be distinguished from another. The skin starts whitening in the beginning and massive round lumps are formed on it. Sometimes this disease affects the eyes and can lead to blindness. In advanced cases of leprosy, the fingers fall off at the joints and the skin over the palms starts rotting. Leprosy is an infectious disease and the patient should be referred to a doctor. The use of products prepared from neem trees are a good remedy for this disease. The body of the leprosy patient should be massaged with a "neem" soap daily, for 45 to 60 days. Neem oil can also be applied on the affected areas of the skin. The body of the leprosy patient should be bathed with water in which leaves of the neem and amaltas trees have been boiled. The leprosy patient should take a salt-free diet and avoid constipation. In general, it is advised that leprosy patients should avoid marriage.

Infection of Red Swelling of the Nail-fold and between Fingers
Chronic paronychia frequently affects housewives. The infection affects nail-folds with a yeast-like fungus called Candida. The condition usually starts in one finger, frequently the middle finger of the right hand, as a glazed red swelling of the nail-fold. Later, other fingers may be involved. Secondary infections caused by bacteria may cause pain and a little discharge of pus

from the nail-fold. Sometimes the nail is lost and the fingers may be disfigured. As the predisposing factor is the prolonged wetting of hands, it is essential to keep hands dry as far as possible to make healing possible.

Whitlow is a term applied to all acute inflammations of the deep-seated tissues in the finger, whether the structure is affected by the root of the nail, the pulp of the fingertips, the skin of fingers or the bone. In this condition, a small painful abscess forms at the base of the nail or the pulp of the finger. Sometimes, the patient feels intense pain as the bursting of an abscess takes a long time. Local application of 1 per cent Gention, violet paint of Mycostatin suspension (P), in the nail-fold twice every day for a prolonged period would help cure the disease. Here is a home remedy : Mix one part of isphagula in four parts of vinegar, and apply to the infected spot. The poulticelike mixture should be bandaged with a clean cloth and water sprinkled over it. The bandage should be changed after every 3 to 4 hours. The inflammation will resolve in 2 to 3 days. Once the pus has been ejected, cooked leaves of neem should be wrapped over the site of the whitlow.

White Marks on Fingernails

White spots on nails are usually caused by slight shocks or pressure to the base of the nail during the time the nail is growing. The spots will eventually grow out but it takes about 3 to 4 months. A full manicure, once a week, is often enough. After that, all that is required is a touch-up through the week — another coat of nail-polish or filing an uneven nail. Frequent removal of nail polish and reapplication of polish can lead to more brittle nails as the powerful nail-polish remover affects the nail.

A weekly manicure is enough for a change of polish. To start with, remove the leftover polish. Shape the nails into an oval curve using an emery board, and then file gently from the outer corners towards the inner areas. Now soak nails in warm soapy water to soften the skin. Clean nails, using a soft nail-brush. To prevent white marks, gently push back the cuticles.

Put cuticle cream around the nail base. Push cuticles carefully with an orange stick with its tip coated in cotton wool.

Rub cuticle massage cream around the nails before going to bed for good results. Always massage hands with a moisturising cream, working down from the wrist to the fingertips and the fingers, then back upwards. Remove grime under the nails with the pointed end of a cuticle stick. Use the stick around the cuticles as well as under the nails. Apply a base coat containing a nail strengthener to clean dry nails. Apply two coats, if polish has not been applied. Brush on the first coat of colour lightly, with three strokes, one down the centre nail, then one on each side. You may prepare cuticle cream by mixing 3 tablespoons of lanolin with the thick tacky fat used in skin foods for a moisturising and softening effect (readily available from dispensing chemists or druggists) and 2 teaspoons China Clay to make it into a paste. There is another simple way to prepare cuticle cream— by mixing half a teaspoon of glycerine with two tablespoons of pure petroleum jelly. Use the mixture on nails as cuticle cream.

Hand lotion is very useful for the rough skin of your fingers and hands. It is available in the market, or can be prepared easily at home. Heat 2 tablespoons of glycerine on medium heat and gradually add cornflour to it so that the mixture thickens. Remove this thick mixture from the heat and add rose water or orange flower juice to it. Keep stirring it for about ten minutes and apply on the skin.

Rough, Tired and Itchy Feet
Rough feet can be tended by dipping them in hot water mixed with a little soda bicarbonate. Scrub the rough parts and heels with a pumice stone. Tender parts like the toes should be scrubbed with a nylon brush. Wipe your feet with a clean, dry towel and sprinkle a good talcum powder on them. The feet have a tendency to sweat profusely, particularly when shoes and socks are worn. They stink and sweat dries the skin. Dry skin should be rubbed with cold cream. Sprinkle some deodorant between the toes and maintain cleanliness by washing socks after each wear. For any swelling, an effective remedy is to massage it with lemon juice or camphor spirit. For itching, wash the feet frequently, dry and then sprinkle powder on them. If knots are there, apply glycerine on the heels and toes and wash off after 30 minutes. Rub honey on the heels before a bath.

4

CARING FOR THE SKIN

Hormones and Their Effect on the Skin
There is a relationship between beauty and hormones. Hormones are produced by the organs in the system of a human body. Lack of hormones or excess of hormones in the body can prove disastrous. Hormones can be introduced in the system by way of pills or injections to regularise imbalance or make up deficiencies. They are of various types, but the ones which are associated with beauty are androgens, estrogens, thyroids, steroids, insulin and sex hormones.

Androgens are basically male hormones but women produce their own androgens in the adrenal gland. If there is excessive secretion of androgens, there will be excessive secretion of sebum of the sebaceous glands, which would cause acne of hair loss. Stress and mental tension may bring about this condition but in such cases the imbalance of hormones may be balanced by taking estrogen pills. Estrogens are normally female hormones produced by the ovaries. They reduce the secretion of sebum, help to cure acne and pimples and benefit the skin by retarding wrinkles and making it clear and shiny. Estrogen pills are essential for women after the age of forty, except for those suffering from high blood pressure. Estrogen therapy sometimes causes harm to the skin, causing pigmentation and skin lesions, and estrogen pills generally lend to a gain in weight. Always follow treatment under medical supervision.

Thyroid hormones are secreted by thyroid glands. If there is a shortage of thyroid hormones in the system the skin becomes dry and wrinkled.

Steroid hormones are produced by the adrenal glands and its excessive production causes skin infections, pigmentation of the skin and acne. Deficiency of insulin hormones harms the complexion and causes skin fungus, becterial infection and itching. Sex hormones are generally of two types : male sex hormones and female sex hormones. Male sex hormones encourage growth of hair on the skin of the body, whereas female sex hormones encourage growth of hair on the scalp.

Caring for the Skin by Electric Therapy
Electricity is a form of energy, which, when in motion, produces magnetic, chemical or heat effects. Before you use electricity for skin care, you should know about the important currents that can be used and their various uses. A galvanic current is a constant and direct current which has opposite poles—a positive pole (anode) and a negative pole (cathode). The positive pole has an acid reaction, soothes nerves, decreases blood supply and hardens tissues. On the other hand, the negative pole has an alkaline reaction, irritates nerves, increases blood supply and softens tissues. The positive pole (anode) may be used to make flabby skin and tissues firmer, to close skin pores after finishing facial treatment, to decrease redness as in mild acne, to prevent inflammation after comedone treatment and electrolysis and to force astringent lotions into the skin. On the other hand, the negative pole (cathode) may be used to remove superfluous hair by electrolysis, to force a bleaching solution into the skin and to stimulate the circulation and nutrition of dry, pale skin and scalp.

A faradic current is an alternating and interrupted current capable of producing a mechanical reaction, without a chemical effect. When a faradic current is applied to the body, the muscles are toned, and the circulation of blood improves. It stimulates hair growth and increases glandular activity. This current may be used during scalp and facial manipulations but do not use this current, in case of pain of discomfort, high blood pressure, broken capillaries or a pustular condition of the skin.

Light Therapy
Light waves travel at a tremendous speed of 1,86,000 miles per second. There are many kinds of light waves, but for beauty and skin care, only three types of rays are important. These are known as ultraviolet rays, infrared rays and visible lights. Infrared rays produce heat whereas ultraviolet rays produce germicidal and chemical reactions.

Caring for the Skin

Ultraviolet Rays

These are invisible rays and their action is both chemical and germicidal. These rays stimulate the activity of body cells and increase iron and vitamin D contents and the number of red and white cells in the blood. The slightest obstruction of any nature whatever will hinder ultraviolet rays from reaching the skin. So the skin must be entirely cleansed before being subjected to ultraviolet rays.

Lamps are available in the market to give ultraviolet ray treatment. If the lamp is placed 30 to 36 inches away, the reaction of the rays will be limited. When the lamp is placed near, within 12 inches from the skin, the rays are not only destructive to bacteria but to the tissues also. Average exposure may produce redness of the skin, and an overdose causes blistering. Always start with a short exposure of two to three minutes and then gradually increase the time to seven to eight minutes. Skin tanning may be the result of one or more exposures to ultraviolet rays, because they stimulate the production of pigment or colouring matter in the skin.

Sunburns occur in various degrees. A slight reddening of the skin are signs of first degree sunburn while itching, burning or peeling are sings of second degree ones. Over-exposure to ultraviolet rays produce third and fourth degree burns which are destructive to the tissues of the skin. Light ultraviolet rays are used for acne, and to combat hair dandruff. They also promote the healing of hair as well as its growth.

Infrared Rays

These rays soothe first degree sunburns. They relax the skin without increasing the temperature of the body, dilate blood vessels in the skin and increase the production of perspiration and oil. To apply infrared rays, the lamp is operated at an average distance of 30 inches. At first the lamp is placed close to the skin, then moved back gradually. Protect your eyes during exposure, and do not permit the light rays to remain on body tissues for a long time. Move the hand, carrying the lamp, back and forth to break constant exposure. The length of exposure should not exceed five minutes.

Visible Lights

The lamp used for reproducing visible lights is usually a dome-shaped reflector in various colours. The blue light has a tonic effect on the bare skin. While the red light has strong heat-rays which have a stimulating effect when used over the skin, it is recommended only for dry and scaly skins. Remember to protect your eyes from the glare and heat of light. Avoid cream, oil and powder to obtain the best results.

Quick Home Facials

The first step in the external care of your skin is cleansing. Perspiration, grease, dust, stale make-up, dirt and bacteria collect on your skin and must be removed completely. Clean the skin with a cleansing cream, milk or lotion or just plain cold cream. Remove the cleanser with tissues, damp cotton wool or a small Turkish towel. Always follow your cleansing routine by toning your skin with a mild skin freshener, a stronger astringent lotion or with a medium strength skin tonic. Toning removes the greasiness remaining from cleansing creams or lotions and closes pores and refines the skin. If you intend to use make-up, it leaves a smooth clean texture which will hold the foundation and powder for much longer.

Nourishing is an essential part of any beauty routine except for very young skin. Dirt, dust, hot and cold weather, cosmetics and even sunlight all tend to dry out the skin, robbing it of moisture and oil. Skin foods attempt to put back some of this nourishment. It is not necessary to use a thick heavy skin food every night. If you do not like to go to bed with a greasy face, it is better to choose a light, easily absorbed skin food which will disappear in minutes. Many of the newer liquid skin foods come into this category. If you feel you need a richer, heavier cream, then use it when you are in the bath.

A facial is the quickest way to revive and liven up jaded skin. It leaves the skin soft, smooth and glowing with vitality. The most luxurious way of having a facial is to go to a beauty saloon where such a thorough job is done that you will that you emerge feeling fresher, looking younger and relaxed. If you get no time or you cannot afford the luxury of regular saloon treatments, then the best thing is to give yourself a facial at home. Choose a quiet time when you are undisturbed. Get the items you need ready before you start so that you can relax and enjoy it. A regular facial once a fortnight is a good habit which will ensure a youthful and fresh skin for a long time. For a quick home-facial, follow these steps:

Caring for the Skin

a) Tie your hair away from the face and neck or wear a bandeau.
b) Cleanse your face and neck with cleansing milk and wipe off, first with a facial tissue and then with a wet towel.
c) Apply cream in dots all over the face and blend it thoroughly - then massage your face and neck in an upward direction.
d) Prepare a face-pack suited to your skin type and apply on your face.
e) When it is dry, wash your face and neck with cold water, keeping your eyes closed. Dry your skin and apply a skin tonic.
f) If you have an important date, use skin tonic after the facial and then apply moisturiser and make-up.

You should choose a face-pack or mask suited to your skin type. Then on a thoroughly clean face, spread a fairly thick layer of the mask of your choice, avoiding the areas of the mouth and around the eyes. Then lie on your back and keep the mask on for 15 to 20 minutes till it dries. Remove the mask with warm water and some absorbent cotton or tissues.

Skin Care by Reflex Therapy

Reflexology, usually called Reflex Therapy or Acupressure Therapy, has become very popular in our country these days. The human body consists of five basic elements : water (*jal*), wood/ earth (*prithvi*), fire (*agni*), air (*vayu*) and space (*aakash*). All these are governed by bio-electricity or life-battery. In order to maintain a proper balance of these elements in the body, we should take food and drink according to the season. Some foods useful in one season can be harmful in another season. For example, buttermilk and curd which are useful in summer are not advisable in the monsoon while fresh vegetables usually beneficial in summer and winter can be a cause of disease in the monsoon because of excessive water content and the possibility of the water being polluted in the monsoon. Similarly, excess of any one of these substances leads to a health problem. For example, colds are very common in winter due to the dampness of air and more water content in foods like rice and fish. The increased incidence of colds means that nature wants to throw out excess water from the body as any retention of it would lead to more diseases. The best cure for the people of a cold country like Japan is to take more food like wheat, have regular sunbaths and drink boiled and lukewarm water. In hot countries like Afghanistan, the fire element predominates in the human body. Dry air, dry fruits and blazing sun lead to excess heat. This can be treated by taking more green, watery fruits like watermelon, avoiding dry fruits in summer and including buttermilk and curd in the diet in greater quantities. Several bodily disorders can be treated and cured by acupressure therapy. Obesity after delivery, greying and falling of hair, pimples, sunstroke, corns and various skin diseases have been cured with reflexology. After childbirth or an operation for sterilisation, women tend to put on weight because of the disturbance of sex glands. Treatment on all points corresponding to the endocrine glands should be undertaken.

Falling of hair and its premature greying is a great problem for women. In such cases, try rubbing of the nails of eight fingers against each other for 10 to 15 minutes every day. It shows wonderful results and may be done for 5 minutes in the morning and 5 minutes before going to bed at night. As soon as the first grey hair is seen, start this rubbing of nails. The hair will remain black for a longer period.

Pimples are sometimes caused by scanty, irregular menses. If there are corns on the feet, massage with ice for 2 to 3 minutes on the affected part. Afterwards, rub turpentine and then bandage the area. By the morning, this corn can be removed. Afterwards, continue rubbing turpentine daily for 2 to 3 days. Rolling the feet on a wooden roller has been found to prevent further formation of corns.

Reflex treatment on the tips of the fingers and toes by vigorous massage and pressing hard on the point below the nose and above the upper lip, helps in treating sunstroke or heatstroke. Symptoms of skin disease are usually due to indigestion and lack of Vitamin 'C', resulting in impure blood. Certain foods mixed and eaten together create poisonous chemical effects in the body and if this poison is not removed from the body by the kidneys, it comes out in the form of eruptions on the skin. It is advisable not to eat cereals, fish, onions, garlic, citrus foods and antibiotics along with unboiled milk, curd and buttermilk. The first urine passed in the morning can be applied on the affected parts to ensure an early cure. Treatment on all points together with more

Vitamin 'C' (*amla*, lemon, fruit juice, raw vegetable) intake and consumption of groundnut and sesame (*til*) in the diet will cure the disease and also remove the problem of dry skin.

Try this health drink which is very beneficial for the treatment of skin disorders. Mix 100 gms of ginger powder in 300 gms of *amla* (gooseberry) powder. Take one teaspoonful of this powder along with water in the morning and evening. Or in four glasses of water, add two teaspoons of the *amla* and ginger powder (fresh *amla* and ginger are better). Now boil the mixture till it reduces to three glasses. Filter the water and drink it. Honey or salt can be mixed in it, if desired. *Amla* is a source of concentrated Vitamin 'C' and has sixteen times more Vitamin 'C' than lemon. Such a drink will give protection to the body against cold and increase its digestive power. People in Western countries drink apple cider which is also beneficial, especially for expecting mothers and growing children. Green vegetable juice is an equally good health drink. Juice made of green spinach (25 gms), *methi* (fenugreek leaves), cucumber, *pudina* (mint), *tulsi* (basil), lettuce, cabbage and coriander is a revitalising drink.

Skin Surgery

Skin surgery is a painful and costly process and has to be carried out only by an experienced surgeon under anaesthesia. There are two important aspects of skin surgery: accidental surgery and plastic surgery.

In case of an accident, the role of the skin is an important point to be considered. If the skin is not given immediate attention, the accidental wound will have many complications. When two layers of ruptured skin are brought together by careful stitches, protection is given to the underlying organs and thus, the body defences come forward like a mother who protects her child in her lap when the child is in trouble. So the point to keep in mind is that in the event of an accident, the skin flaps must be protected to give a healthy cover to the underlying tissues and organs. Within six hours of the accident the wound must be stitched, otherwise the doctor's work becomes more difficult and treatment becomes more expensive for the patient in terms of time and money as well as cosmetically more complicated.

Skin grafting is simply plastic surgery. When the skin is wrinkled, the extra part of the skin is surgically removed and the skin is stitched. Skin grafting, either by free grafts or pedicled flaps, is necessary for optimum healing, and to limit the deformity or disability that occurs when a large area has been lost by injury or burns, disease (varicose ulcers) or by surgical excision of some carcinomas. Free skin grafts provide the simplest method of restoring the skin cover. But they can be used only when the raw surface is composed of healthy vascularised tissues or clean granulations. Ischaemia or infection prevents the healing process.

Split thickness grafts are the ones most generally used though they have a tendency to shrink. They are usually taken from the thigh by means of a special knife. The graft may be affixed by sutures or postage, stamp-sized flaps, and the epithelium grows out from them to cover the intervening bare areas. The proper aseptic precautions are observed for both the grafted area and the donor site (mostly the thigh). A full thickness skin graft, without the fat content, is more effective and gives better colour and texture than the split skin graft. It does not show any tendency to contract and is more useful for the cosmetic areas like the face. But it needs more precautions and better care.

The following medical advice has been given by Dr. Jitender Arora, an eminent skin specialist.

Small Tags of Skin
I often receive queries like the following cry for help:
I am an 18-year-old girl from Rajasthan with a very fair complexion. How do I get rid of the skin tags on my body? During my childhood, when our family was staying in rural areas, tattoos were very popular. These look very odd and shameful now that I am an adult. I feel embarrassed about the way I look. How do I get rid of these skin tags?
Small tags of skin are very common on the neck and in the armpits and groin. They can be removed by tying a fine thread around the stalks so that they drop off. They can be snipped off with sterile scissors or burnt off, but removing them does not prevent more arriving.

Removing tattoos is difficult and unsatisfactory as the tattoo is replaced by a more unsightly scar. Removal must be done only by a doctor, otherwise disasters occur. The tattoos can be removed by cutting them out by Dermabrasion, for example, by replacing the tattoo with discolourd hairless rough skin, by Salabrasion (superficial dermabrasion using salt, by laser) a new, experimental treatment which scars and should be used only in hospitals (and by infrared rays in which very intense heat is applied to the skin) the treatment is quick and simple but leaves scars if done by inexperienced hands.

Baby's Skin Care
It is very important to keep a baby's skin clean at all times, especially in tropical climates where skin infections take long to heal. It is important to use a soap specially formulated for a baby's skin. Use a soft towel and pat the skin dry rather than rub it as rough towels irritate delicate skins. Apply a little baby cream over the baby's skin after drying and before powdering. Fresh air and sunshine are the best tonics for a baby's skin. Sunshine keeps the skin healthy and attractive, but protect your baby's skin from harsh winds by applying baby cream on the cheeks, forehead, nose and chin which will leave an invisible film over the skin. When allowing the baby to sunbathe, always protect the eyes and the back of neck from the direct rays of the sun.

Special care has to be taken in different seasons. In winter, avoid the use of soap and if the skin is oily, use a mild skin tonic. Heavy creams and moisturisers should be used extensively. Use a little vitaminised face cream for skin care. In summer, wash with baby soap at least twice a week if the child's skin is greasy. You may use cleansing milk to clean the skin. In the rainy season, soap should be used once a day and the face washed twice a day with tepid water. An oily skin too needs a moisturiser as a lack of moisture encourages tell-tale lines, even on a child's body.

A massage is a must for a child's delicate skin. Massage with baby oil or olive oil for 10 to 15 minutes before the baby's bath. A sunbathe for a short time is very helpful for a baby's skin.

> *My skin breaks out at the time of my menstrual period. What treatment is advised? While wearing tight-fitting jeans, my daughter gets itchy skin rashes on her thighs and legs. What's the reason?*

Active treatment of the skin, internal treatment with antibiotics, restriction of salt intake, medically supervised therapy to reduce water retention just before menstruation, or possible therapy with hormones may be required to control these breakouts. It is seen that a greater number of skin reactions develop among adolescents who wear trousers with a narrow cut or who wear tight jeans. These include red, itchy and scaling dermatitis, inflamed hair follicles on the front surfaces of thighs and other skin reactions on the thighs and legs. Apart from a red, itchy, slightly scaling skin eruption confined to the body area covered by jeans, there is also an exaggeration in the area covered by the tight trousers, of already existing skin problems. Always wear loose clothes to avoid further skin eruptions produced by pressure or friction and increased heat and humidity caused by a tight fit. Better still, consult your doctor for treatment.

Oils and Your Skin
Every woman wants to be beautiful but while some are born beautiful, others are not. Those who are born beautiful may look worn out with the passage of time and age. This is the reason why, in order to stay beautiful, women of all ages need expert advice, commonly known as Beauty Care. Oils play an important role, and their range is so vast, that they cover the entire range of "Top to Toe" beauty, body and hair treatment. There are a number of oils:

a) Basic or original oils which are pure vegetable extracts.
b) Processed or commercial oils prepared with analytical combinations of various necessary ingredients as required.
c) Synthetic oils have varied uses and a wide range. Almond, coconut, sesame, castor, clove and cinnamon are commonly used varieties of oils available in our country.

The therapy of these oils have not been recommended but prescribed since ancient times in our country. Here is some information regarding the cosmetic and pharmaceutical properties of some oils useful for the skin and scalp.

Almond Oil (Badam)
There are two types of almonds: sweet and bitter. Bitter almonds, contain traces of hydrocyanic acid and are not recommended for beauty care. It oil is used for face massages to improve the complexion and to prevent wrinkles of the delicate skin around the eyes. It is also used to remove eye make-up when the oil is wiped with a wet piece of cotton wool, in a nose to ear direction. For dry and brittle hair, a hot oil massage with almond oil should be given once a week. Oil is useful for a face and body massage when the skin is very dry, in upward and outward directions. In winter, it is applied for heeling chapped lips.

Coconut Oil (Nariyal)

The oil is extracted mostly from the dried kernel which contains about 60-70 per cent oil. Nowadays, oil is also extracted from the coconut shells. Coconut oil with a little camphor has been found to cure skin diseases and wounds. Oil from the shells is used to cure leprosy wounds. For the thickness and growth of healthy hair, apply oil on the scalp with a piece of cotton wool, keep on overnight and wash off in the morning. A massage with coconut oil once a week makes the hair healthy and lustrous.

Sesame Oil (Til Oil)

Sesame seeds are of three types: white, red and black. Maximum oil is found in the white seeds, while the oil extracted from black seeds has medicinal properties. The seeds contain 50 to 60 per cent oil and, therefore, soften rough skins and encourage the growth of hair. It is also the most beneficial oil base in formulations for massages in paralytic conditions. Apply a liberal amount of sesame seed oil to clean facial skin. Massage gently, leaving the eyes and nostrils clear. Now dip a towel in hot water, wring it out, and place over the face for a few minutes to encourage the oil to soak into the skin. Try to lie down with your feet up, to increase blood flow to your face.

Castor Oil

It helps hair growth and since it is thick and sticky in texture, very curly, frizzy and unmanageable hair can be made manageable by combing down with castor oil.

Olive Oil

Olive oil is a good conditioner, excellent for the growth and thickening of hair. Mix two teaspoons of hot oil with henna to make a paste and apply to the hair. Try to leave it on for at least six hours or so and wash it out next morning. Your hair will become glossy and shiny.

5

BODY ODOUR

Every region of the human body has a different odour and sometimes, its origin may easily be identified. There are three important factors which cause odour in the human body:
1) The pattern and type of secretory glands on the skin surface.
2) The positioning of the skin itself. The armpits, for example, make it very difficult for sweat to evaporate and so a characteristic odour is produced.
3) The concentration of bacteria. The number of bacteria are variable in different parts of the body, being maximum in parts like the scalp, axilla, genital areas and the feet.

There are three types of secretory glands on the skin. Sweat glands are the most widely distributed and their function is temperature regulation. The average person loses at least half a litre of sweat every day and this figure rises during the hot season and when physical exercise is done. Sweat has a slightly acrid smell. Areas like the foot pose a problem because the sweat becomes trapped by socks and shoes. The heavy odour associated with the armpits is because the sweat cannot evaporate easily.

There are two other glands, the apocrine and sebaceous glands. The apocrine glands are also a type of sweat glands but they have a limited supply of sweat on the armpits, genital area, nipples and eyelids. Aprocrine sweat is odourless and rich in fats, proteins and other organic materials, all of which make it a breeding ground for bacteria. The bacteria decomposes the sweat to produce the characteristic body odour.

The third type of secretory glands are sebaceous glands and are distributed all over the body, with the exception of the palms and soles. Sebaceous glands secrete an oily lubricant known as sebum which contains cholesterol, fatty acids, waxes and proteins. Sebum is odourless but easily attracts bacteria and these can produce strong odours, particularly around the scalp.

Some parts of the body, like the armpits and genitals have a strong smell because they are richly endowed with all types of glands. Water cannot evaporate from these parts which are usually covered and this leads to offensive body odours. There are millions of bacteria living and multiplying on the skin surface. At the same time, there is always a certain amount of dead matter lying on the surface of the body which provides additional nutrition for the bacteria. Any amount of scrubbing or washing would be able to get rid of only a fraction of the bacteria and that too, for a short while.

Do's and Dont's
1) Use anti-perspirants, deodorants and perfumes available in the forms of lotions, creams, sprays, roll-ons, pads, powders, soaps and sticks. Anti-perspirants contain aluminium salts which close the sweat ducts reducing the release of sweat.
2) Regular baths are a must, three times a day during the summer season being essential.
3) Avoid synthetic wear. Use cotton clothes.
4) Avoid tight-fitting clothes.
5) Avoid hot drinks.
6) Avoid hot, crowded places.

Vaginal Odour : Causes and Cures
A certain degree of distinctive odour is normal in the vaginal area. A traditional and effective method of combating odour here as elsewhere on the body, is cleanliness. Regular soap-and-water cleansing as a part of the normal shower or bath is all that most people require. Body odour is caused by bacteria acting on perspiration, mucus, and sebum (oil) present on the skin, hair and sometimes even on clothes. This may be a special problem on body areas that are normally warm and moist. Feminine deodorant sprays can supplement but not replace cleanliness. If a significant amount of vaginal discharge and/or odour are present, consult a doctor to find the causes.

Sweating Excessively

During the rainy season, are you sweating excessively?

Do you have small red pustules on your body? Do these pustules appear usually on the back, between the folds of breasts, on the neck and the genital area around the vagina?

Do you feel intense itching on affected areas of your body?

Do you feel like scratching the affected parts of your body?

If you say 'yes' to the above conditions, here are some suggestions on how to combat your problem.

Do not scratch the affected skin. It gives temporary relief, but there are chances of the area getting septic. Keep the area dry and clean and sprinkle talcum powder on it. The affected area should be exposed to the open as far as possible. Remember that people suffering from prickly heat should avoid heavy garments and try to expose the affected area to air. Have cold water baths twice every day and follow a few other easy remedies too:

1) Dissolve Fuller's earth *(Multani Mitti)* in water to make a thin paste. It should be smeared over the affected parts. When the paste has dried, wash it with cold water.
2) Apply green henna ground in water on the affected skin.
3) Grind 'neem' leaves in water and apply on the affected skin.
4) The most effective remedy for treating prickly heat is to take a small piece of sandalwood and rub it to a paste on a stone with rose water. Mix in a pinch of powdered alum and apply to the affected skin twice or thrice a week, depending upon the condition of the prickly heat.

A common query is: "I perspire excessively. What do you advise? How can I keep my underarms dry?"

Perspiration is not under voluntary control. Many emotional and environmental factors other than heat influence the quantity of perspiration. Excessive sweating may be related to low-grade infections, internal disorders, other medical problems and menopause. Most anti-perspirants contain some type of aluminium salt that temporarily reduces the transmission of perspiration to the skin surface. None will completely stop perspiration, nor is this desirable, because excessive local dryness would result in severe skin problems. In severe cases, drugs given orally under a physician's care may control excessive sweating, but undesirable side-effects may limit their effectiveness.

No anti-perspirant product will keep your underarms completely dry, especially during brisk walks or during physical activity. The best that can be hoped for is that it will decrease perspiration flow. To stop perspiration completely, sweat ducts must be blocked and this is not desirable as it results in serious skin disorders.

Baths for Skin Care
A bath is an effective beauty therapy. It is important not only for cleanliness but also for the proper maintenance of the skin. If you are using soap, do not use very hot water as it will damage oil glands. Fresh, lukewarm water is best for a bath. Apply soap on the exposed parts of your body to remove dirt and dust particles and do not stint in the amount water you use. Towels should be clean, soft and fluffy. Wipe with a towel by dabbing and then rubbing gently, and do not rub a towel on tender parts like the face, neck, chin and stomach, otherwise wrinkles will appear.

In case of any skin disease, use a medicated disinfectant. In summer, a bath twice a day is essential to wash off sweat and grease, even if some vital materials are destroyed in the process of having a bath. In case of dry skin, the use of soap should be discontinued for a few days. If at all soap is to be used, use glycerine soap, but avoid perfumed or caustic soda soap. Remember, soap is necessary only for cleanliness of the body and not for beauty care. Start soaping the body from the head, then come down to the face, neck, shoulders, underarms, arms, waist, thighs, legs and face. A bath can be taken in running water, standing water, in tubs, under a shower or with steam. Bathing in running water is very beneficial but tub bath is more fashionable than beneficial. When we sit in a tub, all the body dirt dissolves in the water but sticks on to the body again, thus defeating the very purpose of bath cleansing. Bathing under tap water or a shower is good for removing dirt which softens and peels off with the flow of water. It is advisable to apply a sandalwood paste on your body which shall keep the body mildly fragrant and refreshed throughout the day. For this, take sandalwood powder, mix it in rose water to make a paste and then apply a thick coat. Leave it for fifteen minutes, let it dry and then have a bath.

Here is home remedy to lighten a dark complexion: Tie oat flour in a kerchief or a napkin. Dip it in unboiled (raw) milk and rub on the body on alternate days when you have a bath. You will see a miraculous change after a few days. Slowly, the skin acquires a lighter tinge. If you have excess unwanted hair on your body, scrub with gram flour *(besan)* before a bath.

In Western countries, steam baths are very popular and there are public steam bathrooms at many places. In our country, it is becoming popular among people who can afford it though it is not within the reach of ordinary people. More and more health clubs with steam bath facilities are opening as a steam bath is effective for reducing fat, though it has no practical utility as it does not clean the skin. On the contrary, very hot steam may leave an adverse effect on the heart as blood vessels expand permanently due to steam, and sweat glands become overactive.

Sunbathing is very popular in Western countries and men, women and children exposing themselves to the sun on beaches, in hotels and in health clubs is a common sight. In India, however, it is not possible to relax in the sun in public for lack of time, and of course, the traditional narrow outlook! Moreover, since our climate is not cold all through the year, a sunbath is not a necessity.

A Soviet scientist, Nicholas Salus, has established after research that sun-rays affect the white cells the most. For a healthy and clear skin, sun-rays play a significant role. Without exposure to the sun, harmful foreign matter will accumulate under the skin. Sun-rays are also essential for animal and plant life as no plant can grow without the warmth of the sun, no flower can bloom, nor any fruit ripen without it. In a recent experiment when a man was kept away from the rays of the sun for a couple of months, he developed skin abrasions and boils. Sun-rays also give a protective shield to the body which increases resistance to diseases. For pimples and blackheads, sunbathing is recommended. It is good for all skin diseases though long exposure to these rays is harmful and too much exposure to the sun can cause wrinkles and falling of hair.

Breathing and Exercises
Correct breathing is as important to beauty as it is to health, and stimulates the complexion. Air is a free beauty product, so try to make use of it. During the night, always keep the windows open. By simple breathing exercises, you can pull in a sagging stomach, straighten the posture, make the waist slim and even bring a glow to your skin. Also helpful are gentler sports such as walking,

swimming, skating, playing tennis, skiing, rowing, riding and dancing. Gymnastics and aerobics are modern ways of exercises commonly adopted in higher societies.

Cleanliness
In the olden days, we were warned against bathing. We were told that water was bad for the skin. But according to the modern theory the women with the loveliest skin are those who clean their skin regularly. Have a daily bath and wash yourself completely, using plenty of soap and water. People with oily or delicate skins should soften the water with bicarbonate of soda or bran. Use a good toilet or sulphur soap and rub the skin vigorously. A shower is stimulating and reinvigorating and is therefore perfect for the morning. A bath relaxes you and should be taken at night. A warm bath prepares you for sleep and is good for nervous or overweight people. A cold water bath is good for those with flabby muscles and sluggish systems which need a stimulus. You can wash yourself with water at different temperatures on different parts of the body — cold to make the bosom firm, hot to make the ankles slim, etc.

Be careful when applying cold water to breasts. Only douche the tips of the nipples and do it very quickly, as prolonged washing of the breasts could chill mammary glands deeply and cause bronchitis. Many women use ice to rub over the tips of the breasts. The intense cold water causes a very strong static contraction in the mammary muscles without causing a chill.

On a holiday, you should take a 20- minute luxury bath. Make sure that you have the following items :
1) Soft bath towel.
2) Bath cap and hairpins.
3) Friction mitt.
4) Depilatory lotion or cream.
5) Bath-brush.
6) Bath oil or scented bubble bath.
7) Soap and talcum powder.
8) Body lotion or massage cream.
9) Pumice stone.
10) Anti-perspirant spray and scented body cologne.

How to Bathe
1) Pour scented bath oil or bubble bath in the water and run the tap. Do not make it too hot, 75 to 80° F. being hot enough. In the morning, a shower is best. Cold water closes the skin pores and helps you shake off early morning sluggishness.
2) While the tap is running, undress and tuck your hair away from your face and neck. Remove face make-up, if any, with a cleansing lotion. Blow your nose and clean the nostril with a little damp absorbent cotton.
3) Take off your bath robe and get into the bath tub, and relax completely for a few minutes.
4) Now apply soap to the upper part of your body. Rub every part except your breasts with the friction mitt, paying particular attention to your neck. This is usually a neglected area which sometimes becomes grey because of bad circulation. Rubbing with the mitt will help to improve this.
5) Use the friction mitt to give circulation to your upper arms, elbows and shoulders as well as the legs, bottom, heels and ankles. Use a bathbrush to give your back a thorough scrub and prevent spots. Use an anti-perspirant on the armpits.
6) Relax again completely for at least five minutes before stepping out of the bath. Then towel your body dry by patting and rubbing it very gently and apply talcum powder on the underarms, on the feet and on the pubic area with firm, gentle strokes. Rub body lotion or massage cream on the rest of your body. Use both hands to rub it well over your back, bottom, breasts, legs, stomach and arms. Do not forget to wash your eyes and to clean your navel.
7) After your bath, try to relax for few minutes before applying make-up and dressing. After relaxing, if you have time, give yourself a manicure and pedicure before dressing.

6

PREMATURE AGEING

In these days when pollution, dust and smoke makes the atmosphere dirty, a soft, smooth, clear, attractive and glowing facial skin is rare. If you have a good skin, you are blessed. You are the fortunate one. But, mind you, the beauty of your skin will not last long. With advancing age, there is no guarantee that you will maintain that fresh youthful look so you will have to exert yourself to keep it as it is. Normally, worries and tension, coupled with the climatic effect, tell upon the skin and many women look aged even in their prime. Keep up your youthful glow by looking after your skin.

A regular face massage is very essential once a woman crosses the age of 40. A facial massage is an effective way to combat wrinkles. It is a slow process and its results are obvious only when it is continued for a longer period. It is, indeed, not magic which brings a change overnight. There is, however no doubt that a massage reduces unattractive fleshiness, tightens the tissues and muscles and increases blood circulation. It is effective if the skin is clean. After cleansing the facial skin, apply a good cream with light but firm pressure, a process better done with trained fingers which can apply even and firm pressure. With the passage of time, all the visible defects like wrinkles, flabbiness and dead cells vanish and a fresh and young look is restored. A massage should start from the neck upwards and end at the forehead or temples to ensure that all veins and tissues are stimulated for optimum blood circulation. The skin around the eyes is delicate, so it is advisable to apply cream on this part gently. Cream takes 15 to 20 minutes to get absorbed, so massage for that long. Wipe off extra cream with a cotton wool swab

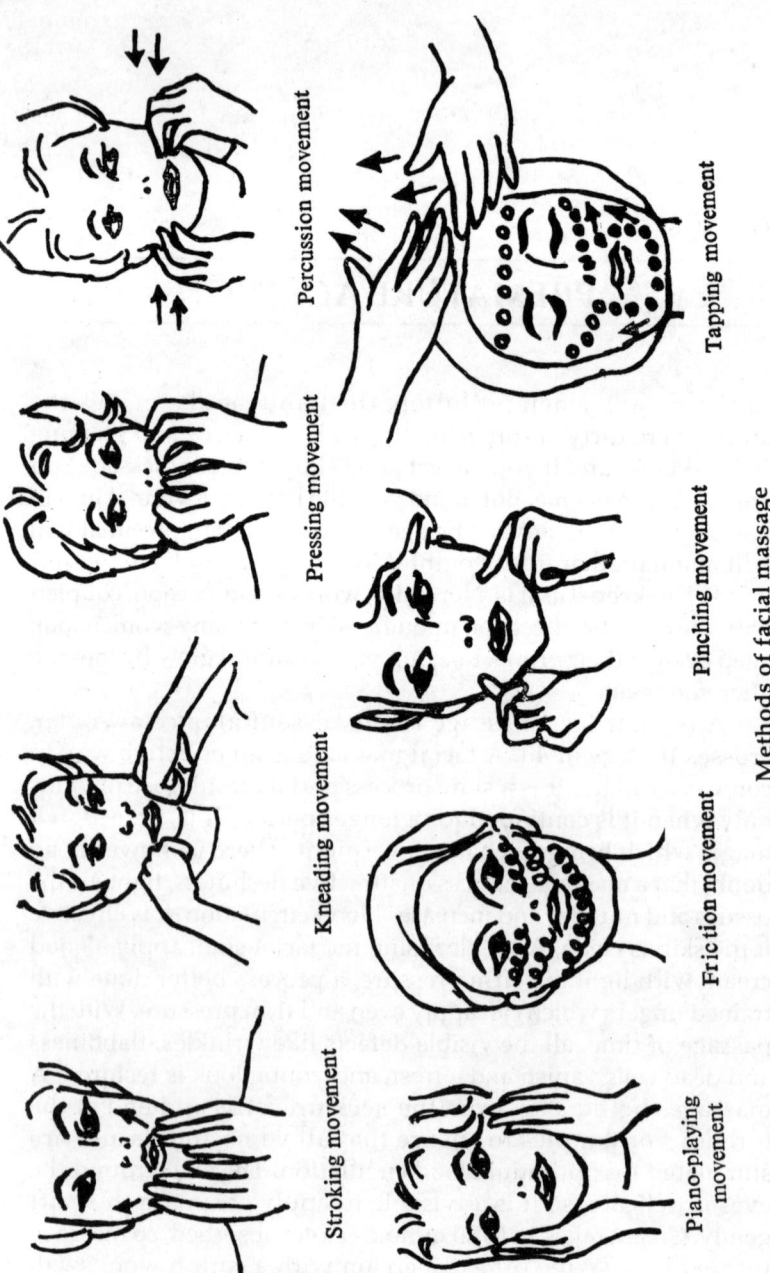

Methods of facial massage

Premature Ageing

soaked in water (preferably rose water). Do not forget to remove all traces of make-up, otherwise the pores of the skin will be blocked by particles of dirt. If there are blackheads, they should be removed. If the skin is oily, apply cleansing milk or pH acid. Fresh lemon juice is also very effective in removing excess oiliness. If the skin is dry, use a good moisturiser before a massage and if the skin is damp, it is advisable to use some astringent lotion. The best time to massage is before going to bed. Apply Vitamin C cream before a massage, but see that the quantity of this cream is enough only to give sufficient greasiness to the skin so that hands and fingers move smoothly on the face. If the face is fleshy and fat, use slimming cream instead of Vitamin C cream.

There are many methods for face massage. A *Slow Massage* is very common and is done slowly by vibrating the skin. The skin is pressed lightly with the soft fleshy tips of the fingers. The process starts with a slow speed from the neck and the speed increases as it moves upwards. Stroking gives rest to the nerves and vibration subdues pain caused by massaging.

A *Fast Massage* is done with both palms to massage with speed. A massage is done with a circular motion upwards.

A *Pressure Massage* is done by applying pressure with the fleshy tips of fingers. This is effective for removing the pouches beneath the eyes.

In a *Stroking Massage*, chubby cheeks are stroked with the tips of fingers. If the nose is broad, strokes are applied from the nose to the temples on both sides of the cheeks.

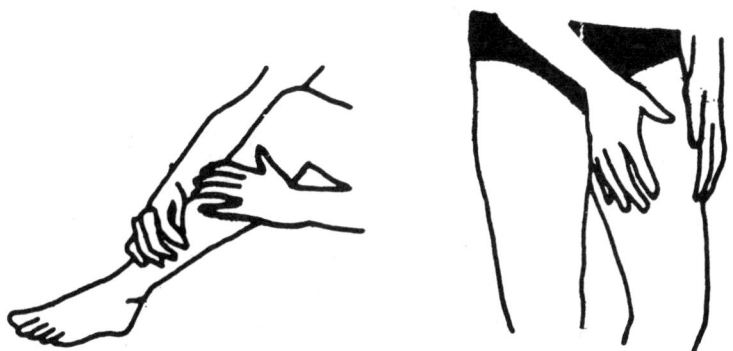

Stroking and deep-stroking movements

In a *Pinching Massage*, the skin is held, as in pincers, between the thumb and fingers. It is effective for double chins and wrinkles of the jaw.

In a *Kneading Massage*, hands are folded in a fist form and the face is pressed as in kneading flour. The movement is made from the chin to the cheeks and upwards. It is good for wrinkled skin.

In a *Friction Massage*, the movement requires pressure on the skin while it is being moved over the underlying structures. The fingers or the palms are employed in this movement. Hand movements are usually employed on the scalp while light movements are used on the face, especially on the neck.

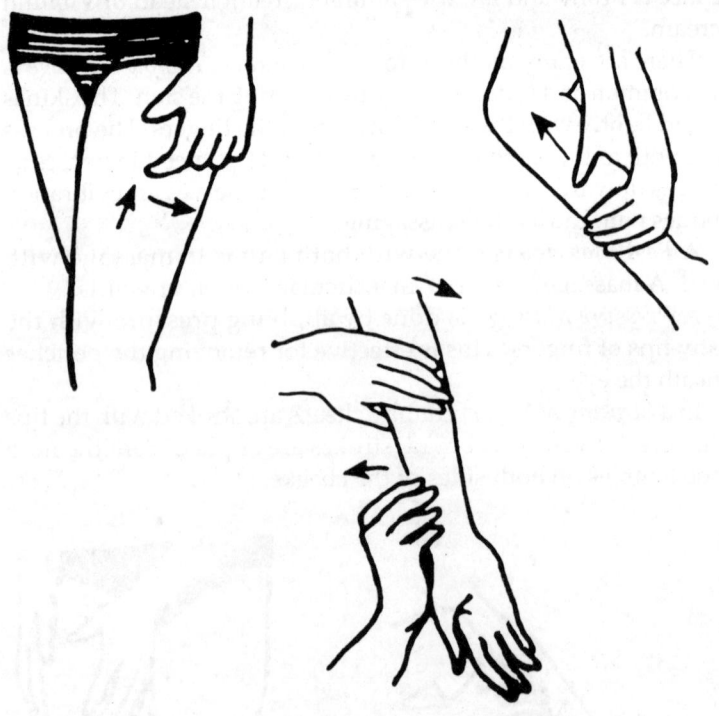

Pinching-Kneading-Friction

In *Piano Playing Movement*, the exercise develops the facial muscles and makes them firm. It should be done over the whole surface of the cheeks with the fingers. The movements must be supple and yet brisk.

Physiological Effects of Massage

To obtain best results from a facial or scalp massage, one must have a thorough knowledge of all the structures involved, such as the muscles, the nerves, and the blood vessels. Every muscle and nerve has a motor point. The position of motor points will vary in individuals due to the difference in body structure. The massage activates circulation, secretion, nutrition and excretion of the skin. Several beneficial results, such as nourishment of skin at all structures, reduction of fat cells in subcutaneous tissues, flexibility and softness of skin, increase in circulation of blood, stimulation of activity of skin glands, strengthening of the skin's fibre muscles, soothing and refreshing of the nerves of the skin are obtained by massage. The frequency of the facial or scalp massage depends upon the age and condition of the skin to be treated. If the skin is in an excellent condition a weekly massage is sufficient.

Remember, when indulging in a facial massage, try to relax, keep silent to maintain a quiet atmosphere, observe utmost cleanliness, make sure your hands are not very cold or warm before touching the skin and the nails of your fingers are not too long or pointed. All self-massage movements must be made in

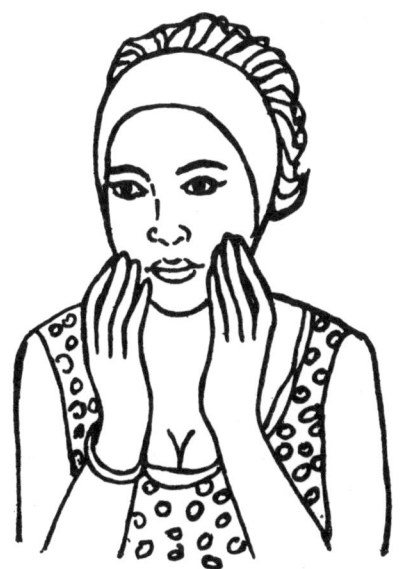

Self-message

the direction of the lymphatic circulation, e.g., towards the heart. When you massage arms or legs, movements must go upwards from the extremities toward the trunk. Do not massage yourself if you are suffering from fever, heart ailment, disorder of the blood vessels, a skin disease, varicose veins, vascular lesions or if you are in the seventh month of pregnancy.

For a Bulging Bottom

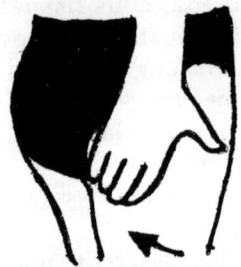

Bottoms are starved of sun and air. Even in summer they are kept covered, and therefore look pale and pasty. Nude sunbathing is not possible in our country, but instead of that you can use an ultraviolet lamp for few seconds every day or have a course of ultraviolet treatment. Always moisturise this area of your body with plenty of body lotion. If the flesh is bulgy and bumpy, do light exercises beneficial for this portion of your body. Pinching the flesh on your bottom when you are in the bath is good for circulation and its shape. Walking provides good bottom shaping. Walking on your bottom will help to reduce bulges and tone up the skin.

7
HIRSUTISM

It must be remembered that unwanted hair, especially on the legs, is actually present in as many as six out of ten women. The basic problem in hirsutism is the excessive action of the male sex hormones, the androgens. An increased amount of androgens may be produced for many reasons, for instance, tumours of the ovaries may be responsible for this. The blood levels of the androgens are then raised above normal. In most women with hirsutism, sometimes the androgen production is not increased, but since downy hair is very sensitive to the low levels of androgens, they get converted into thicker and longer hair.

Heredity and ethnic origin have a lot to do with the amount of hairiness of the skin. Some of the causes of hairy problems are:
1) Mental tension.
2) Effect of medicines.
3) Overweight and infertility.
4) Mild hirsutism may be a normal growing-up process, and a little abnormal hair may appear at puberty or at menopause.

In case the problem is rapid growth of hair and associated with infertility, do consult your doctor.

Can Medicines help reduce Hairiness?

Treatment of hirsutism depends on the cause as well as on its severity. The cause needs to be determined by examination and investigations like X-rays and ultra-sonograms. However, sometimes specialised investigations like estimations of blood levels of androgens, specialised X-rays and even a laproscopy may be required (Laproscopy is a process in which visualisation of abdomen is carried by using a tube). After the cause is established, it needs to be treated.

What to do for Excessive Hair on Face and Body
Excess hair, particularly on the face, is a matter of great concern to a woman. There can be many reasons for this unwanted growth, like congenital causes, imbalance of hormones, pregnancy, irregular menses, mental tensions, long illness, worries and shocks. One should immediately rid oneself of unwanted hair when it starts growing, instead of feeling shy and embarrassed. In medical terminology, this condition is called Hirsutism. Unwanted hair grows mostly on the chin, above the upper lip and on the forehead. Most of the women suffering from hirsutism are in the age group of 15 to 25. Since the main reason for the growth of unwanted hair is imbalance of hormones inside the body, it is imperative to get it treated medically. The first step in the medical treatment is a thorough check-up of the genitals. In case of some defect in the uterus, it is treated by an operation. There are many ways to get rid of a thick growth of hair such as shaving, plucking, threading and waxing. Electrolysis is the only permanent treatment for removing facial hair, but being costly, this treatment is beyond the means of women of the middle-income group.

Usually, people ask many question about superfluous hair and some of the very common ones are as follows.

What is Hirsutism and what are Its Causes?
Most, if not all, adult males have visible hair growing on their faces and body. Women, on the other hand, have only very fine downy, inconspicuous hair on the face and body. If hair becomes darker, thicker and visible, then the woman is suffering from hirsutism, a problem that may cause intense misery. Consult a skin specialist and remember that medicines should be taken strictly with the consultation of a doctor. Medication may prove very useful when used alongwith cosmetic treatment, reducing the growth of hair and finally with continued treatment, making the hair inconspicuous.

How does one get rid of Superfluous Hair Cosmetically?
Hairy legs may upset a female but it need not cause worry. You may get rid of this problem by cosmetics or home-made preparations. What you can do about it depends on the time and money you want to spend. If it is necessary to remove the hair, depilation or epilation are the time-honoured methods.

Hirsutism

Depilation removes the hair at skin level or sometimes just below the skin level. Epilation, on the other hand, removes the full length of hair.

a) Plucking-threading

If there are one or two unwanted hairs on the face, then it can be pulled out by a tweezer. This method is known as plucking. If there is a lot of hair, then do not use a tweezer, because the roots of the hair get hardened and the repeated pulls may result in injury to the roots and subsequent growth of pimples and acne. Before using a tweezer, apply cold cream on the area to soften the roots. In case the roots are hard, then soak a swab of cotton wool in hot water and keep it on the hair for some time. This will soften the roots. When thread is used to remove hair, the process is called threading. Threading does not make the roots of hair hard. It should be done after two or three weeks. Never use a razor to remove the hair. It hardens the roots of hair and also encourages rapid regrowth of hair.

b) Shaving

Shaving is an unacceptable method of dealing with facial hair among women in our country. At the same time, it is probably the most commonly used method of dealing with superfluous hair on the legs and underarms. It is a total fallacy that hair grows faster and becomes coarser after shaving. Of course, the hair does reappear with great rapidity, but this is not because hair growth has been stimulated, but because shaving cuts the hair just at the surface, leaving the hair with blunt tips. Another disadvantage with shaving is the risk of nicking the skin. This can be reduced by using a swivel-head razor. For best results, use a sharp blade razor slowly and carefully. Electric razors give best results, though the initial investment is expensive. Wetting the hair makes shaving easier and soaping keeps the hair wet for a longer time. Remember, avoid using an anti-perspirant or a deodorant for at least 10 to 12 hours after shaving.

c) Using a Pumice Stone

Abrasives, in the form of pumice stones and special emery covered mitts and pads, are frequently used to remove superfluous hair.

This method is very cheap and its effects are very temporary. But it is good for the skins which tend to suffer reaction quickly.

Use gentle circular movements and apply a moisturising cream after the use of abrasives. If the skin is rubbed too vigorously, it will become tender and sore. This method is used for coarse hair of the legs and arms, and is not suitable for use on the face. After waxing, the regular use of pumice stone can delay the regrowth of hair.

d) Waxing

Waxing is the most useful and one of the oldest methods of removing unwanted hair, but it should be only used for removing hair from the hands, arms and legs. By waxing, the skin of the face gets stretched, resulting in wrinkles. The wax used is usually of two types : cold and hot. A cold wax can be used without being heated. It is readily available in market, but is expensive. You may prepare home-made wax yourself.

Take eight parts of sugar syrup and add one part lemon juice, one part mustard oil and two parts water. Brew it on medium heat for about 45 minutes. When the mixture turns brown in colour, remove it from the flame and add a little glycerine. Let it cool. Honey can also be used to make hot wax. For this take five spoonfuls of honey, and add one spoonful of lemon juice and heat for 30 minutes on a medium flame. Remove it from the heater and add a little glycerine.

Waxing is a method commonly used in beauty parlours. The skin must be cleansed by a cleansing cream before waxing. You must use unheated milk in case cleansing cream is not available. A creamy milk should not be used because it further accentuates the growth of unwanted hair. Use a clean towel to wipe the skin, and while spraying talcum powder, massage it very gently. If the thick roots of hair cause pain, then use cold cream for massage before waxing. This will soften the roots.

Apply hot wax on the skin with a knife towards the direction of the growth of hair. Use a thin cloth as a bandage on it so that the cloth sticks to the skin. Now pull the cloth with a jerk in opposite directions of the roots of hair. The hair will stick to the cloth and come out with the root. The container of wax should be kept in another utensil full of warm water so that the wax remains hot and melted during the process. Waxing should preferably be done in an air-conditioned room or under a fan, otherwise the wax will not stick to the hair due to sweat. Even a cooler does not help as the moisture from it prevents proper waxing.

Immediately after waxing, the skin should be lightly massaged with lanolin-cream or a skin tonic. This will make the skin smooth and silky.

e) Chemical Depilation

Depilation is the method commonly used for removing superfluous hair on the arms, legs and underarms. Specialised preparations have now been produced by certain cosmetic manufacturers for exclusive use on the face. Depilatories are generally thioglycollate-based and sulphide-based. They weaken the hair protein—keratin—by reducing the hydrolysis in an alkaline pH. The hair breaks just below the skin surface. The time required for depilation depends on the coarseness of hair, varying between 5 to 15 minutes. Use of soluble alkalis, like sodium hydroxide, reduces the depilation time. Depilatory agents are available as creams, lotions and sprays (Aerosol spray are the latest methods of applying depilatories). Lotions are easier to apply over a larger surface. Irritation and dryness of the skin may occur, because the chemicals act on the keratin of the skin, dryness becoming evident after about 24 hours. To counter the dryness, two-stage products are available in the market. The second stage emollient soothes the skin and enhances the smoothness of the skin. It is buffered at acidic pH to ensure the neutralisation of any residual alkali. A similar effect can be achieved by swabbing the area with a home-made neutralising solution.

Mix one part lemon juice or vinegar to seven parts of cold water and apply immediately after the depilatory cream has been removed, followed with an application of cold cream. Remember not to use depilatories on broken skin, since it may develop an allergic reaction.

f) Bleaching Superfluous Hair

Bleaching is one way of making existing hair less conspicuous and is good for down, rather than for thick coarse hair. It is the most commonly used method for camouflaging facial hair. A simple bleaching system consists of hydrogen peroxide containing ammonia to give a pH of 9 to 10. Bleaching is also very useful in revitalising the paleness of the skin due to heat, dryness and superfluous hair and prevents growth of unwanted facial hair. It colours the thin and fine hair and keeps the complexion fair by hiding these tiny hairs. Waxing sometimes causes wrinkles and threading hardens the roots of hair, thus bleaching has been considered the safest process by leading cosmetologists. The only problem with bleaching is irritation, which happens either when too much ammonia has been used or when the bleach is kept on for long periods. The reaction usually subsides after a few hours. When the reaction is severe, seek your doctor's help. You may go for a skin test, if your skin is too delicate. Apply bleach on a delicate part and observe its reaction for sometime. If the skin feels itchy, avoid going for a bleach. Do not bleach, in the following conditions:

1) During menstruation.
2) During pregnancy.
3) After childbirth, if the baby is breast-feeding.
4) If your skin is too sensitive and delicate.
5) If you are suffering from some skin disease.
6) If you have asthma, heart or kidney trouble.
7) If you feel a burning sensation when bleaching.

g) Electrolysis

Electrolysis, as a means of permanently removing unwanted hair, was introduced by Dr. Charles Michael in 1857. In the year 1916, this treatment acquired prominence among the various methods of enhancing the beauty. In this process, the roots of hair are weakened by subjecting them to electric currents and repeated treatment stops their growth. There are two methods of electrolysis to burn the hair. One is the "Galvanic multiple needle method" and the other is the "short-wave method". In India, the short-wave method is much in vogue. A single needle is used to remove hair by this method. Remember, always go for this treatment to a qualified and experienced beautician only. In order to make the area insensitive or dead, Zylokin is rubbed as an anaesthesia and then the slanted needle is pricked to reach the root of the hair, the thickness of hair deciding the depth of the needle. Then the roots of the hair are burnt by using electric currents. Electrolysis should not be used to remove hair from eyelashes, the inner side of the nose and ear or from pimples.

Do not go for electrolysis in case:
1) You are suffering from diabetes.
2) You are being treated by a doctor for hormone deficiency.
3) You have a pimply skin.
4) You suffer from skin problems.

Precautions for Using Electrical Devices

Like the Galvanic needle which is used for electrolysis, there are several other electrical appliances used to treat the skin and scalp. The vibrator is an electrical appliance used in a massage to produce a mechanical succession of manipulations. It has a stimulating effect on the muscular tissues, increases blood supply to the parts to be treated, is soothing to the nerves, increases glandular activities and stimulates the functions of the skin. The vibrator is used over heavy muscular tissue such as the scalp, shoulder and upper back. Avoid the use of a vibrator on facial tissue. People suffering from fever or a weak heart should avoid the use of a vibrator.

A steamer is an electrical device used to produce a moist, uniform heat. It is used to cleanse and steam the face, clean out the pores of the skin and soften any horny scaliness on the surface of the skin. A heating cap is another device, applied over the head, to produce a uniform source of heat. It is used to recondition dry, brittle and damaged hair and also serves to activate a sluggish scalp. Hair dryers deliver hot, medium and cold air for proper drying of the hair. You must observe the following precautions when using electrical devices:

1) Disconnect the appliances when not required for use.
2) Keep all wires, plugs and equipment in safe conditions.
3) Safeguard against cords getting wet and do not handle a device with wet hands. Do not clean the appliance when it is plugged in.
4) Sanitise all electrodes properly. Do not touch a metal while using an electrical appliance. Do not touch two metallic objects at the same time while connected to an electric current.

A young college student asks

I have coarse, dark hair on my legs and feel most embarrassed when wearing swimsuits or bikinis and short dresses. I am a young girl around twenty usually wearing skirts. Is it possible to get a permanent relief by electrolysis?

No. I will not suggest electrolysis for removing leg hair. This treatment is quite costly. The way you deal with leg hair depends on the coarseness. Bleaching, shaving, depilatory creams and waxing are some of the methods to get rid of superfluous hair on the legs.

Bleaching works well for fair, downy hair if the growth of hair is short and fine. In hot weather you will find that the hair growth becomes fairer in the sunshine, so the bleaching process will not be necessary very often. Bleaching weakens the hair too. I will not suggest shaving on the legs. The disadvantage is that the regrowth is stubbly and rough, regrowth of hair is too rapid. There is the danger of cutting the skin, particularly over the shinbone. Depilatory creams give a smooth finish on the legs but must be used twice a week for lasting results. Apply the cream all over the hairy area, wait for about five minutes, then remove the cream with a spatula. Next, wash or shower in lukewarm water and then rub in some moisturising cream as the depilatory cream is very drying. The process is a bit costly. Depilatory creams in aerosol form are more convenient to use, but they are uneconomical. Waxing is a good answer to the problem of dark, tough hair, as the results last for about five weeks. However, it is fairly painful, so try it first at a beauty parlour. If the discomfort does not worry you, it's most easy to do and in an economical method.

8
HEALTHY HAIR

The scalp is nothing but the skin on the head. The skin of the scalp is similar to the skin elsewhere on the human body and like the skin, consists of two layers : the dermis and the epidermis. However, large and deeper hair follicles are present on the scalp to accommodate the longer hair of the head.

The hair is composed of a protein called keratin. The chemical composition of hair is:

Carbon	:	50.56%
Hydrogen	:	6.38%
Nitrogen	:	17.14%
Sulphur	:	5.00%
Oxygen	:	20.85%

The chemical composition varies with the colour of the hair. Full grown hair is divided into two parts : the root and the shaft. The rate of hair growth varies from person to person. The average growth of hair is approximately 1/4 inch per month, i.e., 1/16 inch per week. The growth of hair is always greater between the ages of 20 and 30 and faster in summer than in winter. The growth of hair is cyclical, i.e., after a few years of growth, the hair enters a phase of inactivity, then dies and falls. A hair dies when its bulb is separated from the papilla that feeds it. The hair bulb is a thickened club-shaped structure forming the lower part of the hair root. The lower part of the hair bulb is hollowed out to fit over and cover the hair papilla. The papilla is a small cone-shaped elevation found at the bottom of the hair follicle that fits into the hair bulb. Within the papilla is a rich blood and nerve supply, which contributes to the growth and regeneration of the hair. Through the papilla, the nourishment reaches the hair bulb.

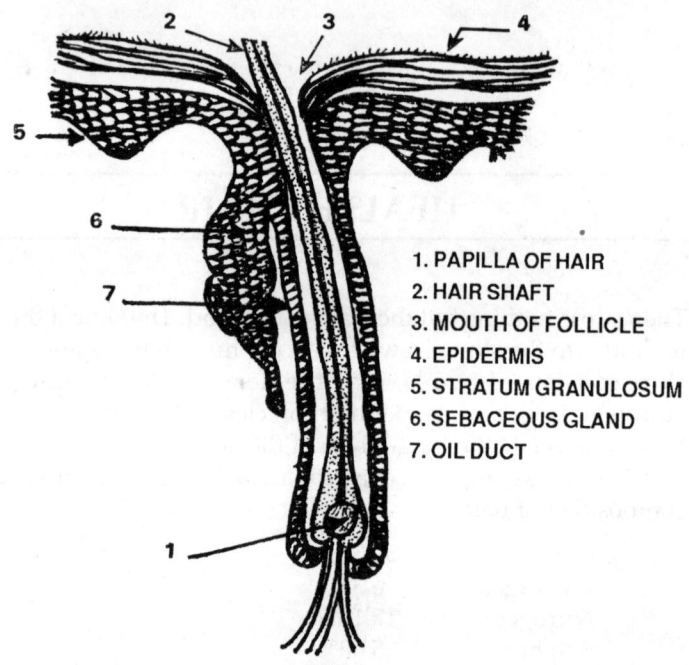

A cross-section of the scalp

1. PAPILLA OF HAIR
2. HAIR SHAFT
3. MOUTH OF FOLLICLE
4. EPIDERMIS
5. STRATUM GRANULOSUM
6. SEBACEOUS GLAND
7. OIL DUCT

The growth of the scalp hair occurs rapidly between the ages of 15 and 30, but declines sharply between 50 and 60. Scalp hair grows faster in women than in men. A certain amount of hair is shed daily. The average daily shedding is estimated at 50 to 80 hairs. Hair loss beyond this estimated average indicates some scalp or hair trouble. Eyebrow hair and eyelashes are replaced every 4 to 5 months.

The average life of a hair will range from 2 to 4 years. Factors such as sex, age, type of hair, heredity and health affect the duration of its life. The average area of a head is about 420 square inches and there is an average of 10,000 hair per square inch. The number of hair on the head vary with the colour of the hair, and the colour of hair, whether it is fair, brown or black, depends on natural pigment on its cortical cells—melanin. Melanin is

Healthy Hair

produced in the pigment cells of the bulb and then passed into the cells of the cortex.

Home-made Herbal Hair Tonic

Melt 2 tablespoons lanolin, 3 tablespoons castor oil, 1/2 tablespoon coconut oil and 1 teaspoon glycerine. Now add 1/2 cup water, continuously beating until thoroughly mixed. Now add 1 teaspoon each vegetable lard, vinegar and liquid soap. Make it more nutritious, by adding an egg.

Baldness among Men and Women

Male baldness runs in families and is due to male hormones. It starts after puberty over the temples and the hairline which recedes, resulting in a high forehead. The top of the scalp loses all the hair and become smooth. Usually, women lose hair as they grow older. Eczema of the scalp also lead to baldness in some cases.

Dandruff

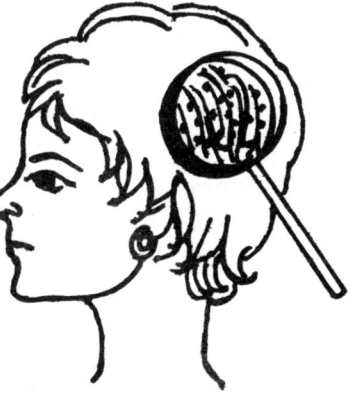

Poor circulation of blood, poor hygiene and an improper diet are are some of the causes of dandruff. Dandruff is of two types: Dry dandruff (which is also known as pityriasis capitis simplex in medical term) and Waxy dandruff (pityriasis steatoides). Dandruff is generally believed to be infections. From the cosmetologist's point of view, both forms of dandruff are to be considered contagious and may be spread by the use of common brushes, combs, towels, soaps and other articles. Take necessary precautions to clean and disinfect everything that comes in contact with the hair. Dry dandruff is characterised by an itchy scalp and small white scales usually attached to the scalp or loosely scattered in the hair. The waxy or greasy type of dandruff accuse when the scaliness of the epidermis is mixed with sebum which causes it to stick to the scalp in patches. The itchiness causes the person to scratch the scalp. If the greasy scales are torn off, bleeding or oozing of sebum may follow.

Medical treatment is advisable for this condition. If there is the slightest sign of dandruff, treat it without delay. There are a number of excellent preparations available in the market for curing it. Two simple household remedies to fight dandruff are described below:

1) Mix two tablespoons of cosmetic vinegar and six tablespoons hot water. Dab with cotton into the scalp, parting the hair with a comb. Preferably, apply it at bedtime and tie a scarf over the head to avoid staining the bedclothes. Next morning wash the hair with a shampoo. After the hair is thoroughly rinsed, pour over as a last rinse, a mixture of 3 tablespoons of cosmetic vinegar and a cup of hot water.

2) Hot oil therapy is another method to cure dandruff. Massage hot oil into the scalp at bedtime. Next morning, an hour before the bath, rub lemon juice mixed with cosmetic vinegar into the scalp with cotton wool. Give the hair a good wash with egg shampoo. As a last rinse, use the juice of one lemon in a cup of hot water. Continue this treatment once or twice a week for three months.

Giving the hair and scalp a hot steam bath is useful. Massage hot oil and wrap a hot damp towel on the head like a turban, so that the steam can fight dandruff.

Patchy Baldness

The sudden appearance of small bald circles on the female scalp may seem like a world shattering event. It is even more alarming

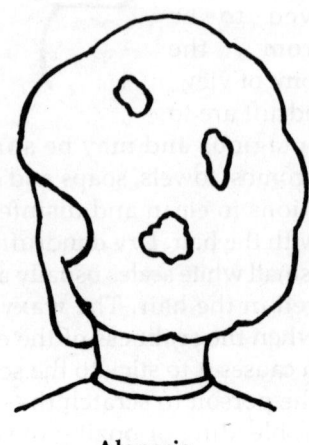

Alopecia

if these patches grow larger and join up. The causative factors of baldness are almost the same as those which contribute to premature greying of hair. It may be due to serious disease, anaemia, great anxiety or sudden shock. Premature baldness is generally hereditary and it is difficult to cure. Eczema of the scalp also leads to baldness in some cases. If the baldness is due to any serious disease, a naturopathic cure will be beneficial. The drugs recommended for premature greying would help to check falling of hair also but consult your doctor for this. Once the hair has fallen and the follicles have closed, nothing can be done. There are a few home remedies for patchy baldness. Preserve mangoes in oil for a period of one year and rub this oil on the scalp.

Another home-remedy is to grind the remains of tobacco in a hookah in mustard oil and use it for massaging the scalp.

Alopecia is the technical term for any form of loss of hair. The natural falling of the hair should not be confused with alopecia. In natural falling of hair, these patches nearly always regrow after six to twelve months without any treatment. The new hair is often white but later becomes the normal colour. The hair lost in alopecia does not regrow, unless special treatment is given to encourage hair growth. Alopecia is not infectious. Some medical authorities believe it to be caused by a disturbance of the sympathetic nervous system. Alopecia is a particular type of baldness in patches and with proper treatment, the bald patches again grow hair, but it takes months for the full growth. Steroid tablets produce regrowth of hair in patches, but it has been observed that hair falls out again. Local injections of steroids and strong steroid applications smay accelerate regrowth but to do so may cause thinning and pitting of the scalp. Producing an allergic eczema on the scalp using chemicals or plant extracts, may work, but they have to produce a severe eczema. Research is going on for a solution. One must consult a skin specialist for allopathic treatment. Alopecia is generally of three types: *Alopecia senilis* which usually occurs in old age, where the hair loss is permanent; *Alopecia premature* is the form of baldness beginning any time before middle age by a slow thinning process; and *Alopecia aerata* is the sudden falling of hair in round patches or baldness and may happen even at a young age.

Greying of Hair

Every time you pull a grey hair, ten more grey hairs will come out—so remember never to pull a grey hair but instead, cut it near the root. Temporary rinses are less in use and not in vogue. Hair dyed with herbs are difficult to set, so people are more inclined towards chemical dyes. These cannot produce drastic changes in hair colour.

In case, you have a lot of grey hair use chemical hair dyes. This is a very popular dyeing method in our country. The dye is more or less permanent and if dyed well, hair looks almost a natural black. Dyes are not affected by the climate, season, water and soap. The dyes are made with chemicals like para, hydrogen peroxide and others, and are easily available in the market.

For dyeing, wash your hair clean, remove all grease and apply the dye as per instructions with a brush. Dye leaves a black colour on fingers and nails which may mar the beauty of hands. So use rubber gloves. Do not apply the dye on the skin of your scalp (apply on hair only). Let the dye remain on the hair for about an hour, then wash it off with shampoo. Dyeing is to be repeated after a fortnight or so, because when the hair grows, roots start showing grey again. The chemicals used in dyes sometimes causes a reaction on the skin. It may cause a burning sensation immediately after applying or can take up to 48 hours to occur. Reddishness starts with the ears, spreads to the eyes and then the whole face swells. Eczema may also erupt. It is, therefore, advisable to take a skin test by applying some dye behind the ear or the neck where the skin is very sensitive. The test can be done on the inner part of the elbow where the skin is tender. If there is no reaction within 48 hours, go ahead with using the dye. But, there is no guarantee that you are immune to reaction forever. It is better to test every time before the dye is to be used.

In case of a reaction on the skin, consult a doctor and take the prescribed medicine. In order to ward off the ill-effects of para-chemicals, use water with sodium chloride to clean your hair. This mixture is made like this:

Take two litres water, two tablespoonfuls of sodium chloride and one tablespoonful of hydrogen peroxide. Mix these and wash hair twice a day. It is, however, necessary to consult a doctor in case of any skin abrasion or reaction. If a doctor is not available, take one of the following solutions and apply it on the skin with a handkerchief.

Take fresh clean water. Add boric powder to it and apply on the affected part. Another way is to take 10 camomile flowers and put them in boiling water. Strain and apply on the affected skin. Remember, do not dye the hair in case conditions, such as menstruation, pregnancy, asthma, heart problem, kidney trouble, skin diseases, breast-feeding, extremely dry hair or fall of hair prevails. If you feel a burning sensation while dyeing, stop operations immediately and have a skin test.

Premature greying or falling of hair signifies some deficiency of the body. The quality of hair depends upon the general health. A polluted atmosphere, scorching heat, humid climate affects the beauty of the hair adversely. Likewise, tension, anxiety, grief, disease, frustration or brooding are also harmful. To make dry hair look shiny and healthy, try a soft massage with warm oil.

Dry, Brittle and Dull Hair

The first imperative to manage hair is a daily scalp massage, using circular motions and making sure that fingernails do not dig in and damage the scalp. Shampoo every week, and after each wash, to detangle, soften and eliminate static electricity. Use a cream conditioner to heal dry, damaged hair by filling in crevices and smoothing the surface. Dry, dull hair responds well to oil treatment. Massage warm oil into scalp and wrap your hair in a hot, wet towel for ten minutes before shampooing.

If the hair looks dry, dull, lifeless and does not fell silky, the causes my be that it has lost its natural barrier of oil and moisture when it has been over-processed or over-shampooed. Exposure of hair for two long to the sun and wind, and chlorination due to salt water can damage the hair. In this case, use a low detergent shampoo formulated for dry hair in small quantity. Always finish with a moisturising conditioner. Let your hair dry naturally. If you want to use a hair dryer, hold it at least six to eight inches away from your head and keep it moving. As regard continuous use of a hair dryer, the heat from it will not affect your hair, even if you use it every day, provided you keep it on the low or comfort cycle. Do not keep the dryer pointed at one spot too long, but keep it continually moving on your head. Using a dryer on a very hot cycle may cause flaking of the scalp if the hair is oily—in fact, the new comb-through dryers just dry the hair, not the scalp.

Hair Conditioning

Conditioners are to hair what moisturisers are to skin. They give lustre and body, make it more manageable and help replace oils and proteins. There are three basic types: *Instant conditioners, Body-building conditioners,* and *Corrective conditioners.* Instant conditioners help manage hair that does not hold a set. They work by coating hair with beneficial conditioners and depositing protein to help fill the hair-shaft. Body-building conditioners add bulk to fine, sparse hair. Each strand becomes coated with conditioners and plumps it in diameter, to give the effect of hair that is fuller and thicker. The corrective conditioner helps repair the hair damage with connectants, to relieve dryness and add shine and protein to restore natural elasticity and help make hair more supple and resistant to damage.

The right way to shampoo hair is to start by liberally wetting your hair with warm water and then massaging lather in your scalp. Give special attention to the crown and sides of the head, which are often neglected, follow with a long, thorough rinse—atleast two minutes—flooding the water through the hair. Repeat it if necessary, but if you shampoo your hair every day, one application is sufficient. Water temperature should start at warm and taper off to cool or cold, if you can stand it. Cold water seems to close pores and bring a shine to hair.

Brushing provides strength and lustre to the hair, but excessive brushing is harmful. In case, your hair falls out in clumps, there may be several causes—serious illness, sudden hormonal changes, mental tension, running a very high fever, or a deficiency of important nutrients in the diet. To cure such type of hair loss, brush hair gently with a soft, natural bristle brush. Do not pull or twist your hair. Shampoo lightly with a mild shampoo. Avoid the use of blow-dryers or hot rollers. Salt and chlorinated water make the hair hard and sticky. Also, if the hair has been coloured, they tend to bleach the colour out. Always wash your hair immediately after swimming in salt or chlorinated water. If you can't shampoo, rinse with soda water. In case, you have only little grey hair, apply henna and avoid use of chemical hair dyes as far as possible.

Pediculosis—Lice Infestation

Any slackness in cleaniness breeds lice infestation. A louse is a parasitic insect with six clawlike feet. It is grey in colour but it turns brownish after sucking blood, which it does with two small trunklike whiskers. A louse egg hatches in nine days and within a fortnight, the young ones attain maturity. Long hair is more prone to lice infestation. The back of the head itches when infested with lice, and itching causes abrasion of the scalp skin. Lice can be controlled by removing their eggs in the initial stages. Avoid using towels, soap or comb of a person who has lice.

Nits (lice on the scalp) cause havoc in schools where lice infestation is common. The adult lice runs from one scalp to another, sticking eggs on the hair with a strong cement-like substance. The pearly nits look like sticky dandruff, but cannot be shaken off. Running a nail along the hair will not detach the eggs. The scalp infestation by lice indices scratching which in turn may cause bacterial infection. The insect lays eggs which are contained in a whitish ovoid receptacle called the nit, which is attached to the hair by a collar. The nit can be slid along the hair but not pulled off. The search for lice or nits in suspected cases of pediculosis of the scalp should be made on the back and sides of the head.

The lice can be killed with a single application of 1 per cent gammabenzene hexachloride, or 2 per cent DDT emulsion or 25 per cent benzyl benzoate emulsion. The scalp should be washed after 24 hours, and the nits should be carefully removed with a comb as the ova are unaffected by these agents. The treatment may have to be repeated after a week or ten days. You may consult a doctor also.

Body lice (pediculosis corporis) reside in the seams of clothing and not on the skin surface. The clothes should thus be treated with a thorough powdering of 10 per cent DDT powder or should be boiled for 10 to 15 minutes. The itchy skin lesions respond to soothing agents like calamine lotion, which should be applied after a hot bath. There are a few ways for controlling lice:
1) An anti-lice oil can be mixed with coconut (or mustard) oil and 0.2 per cent lindane (BHC) or 0.1 per cent prethrum essence. This oil can be rubbed well into the scalp to kill lice. (Ingredients can be purchased from a chemical dealer).
2) Mix talcum powder with 0.2 per cent prethrum dust in it (or add 10 per cent DDT). Sprinkle this powder on the hair before going to bed and rub it vigorously so that it reaches

the roots. Cover your mouth, nose and eyes to protect them from the powder.

3) Anti-louse lotion, either gammabenzene hexachloride lotion or cream (Lorexane, Gammaexane) or malathion (Prioderma) will kill the eggs which can be removed by a comb with very fine teeth. One treatment is enough but all the family who are infested should be treated and the hair examined regularly for a while. You may consult a doctor for the treatment.

The above-mentioned concoctions should be used at night. Tie a cloth around your head after applying any one of the medicines, let it remain at least for 24 hours. Before washing off, do not use soap or shampoo. Repeat this for a week and lice and their eggs will be eliminated. Pediculosis pubis refers to infestation by a crab-shaped louse. In addition to the pubic area, it also affects the armpits, legs, hairy chest, eyebrows and the eyelashes.

9

BEAUTY OF THE BREASTS

No other part of a woman's body is so attractive as her breasts which add to the overall beauty, charm and grace of a woman. The first thing that attracts an onlooker is the bustline of a passing woman.

Breasts are basically made up of cells, glands, tissues, milk ducts, fibrous tissue and fat. There are no muscles in the breast tissue. A buxom and full breastline is a symbol of feminine beauty. A female becomes aware of the beauty of her breasts as soon as she steps out of her adolescence and attains youth. Although, shapely breasts are the gift of nature, their maintenance is in your own hands. Timely care since early adolescence, when a woman is in her formative years, can help her in keeping her breastline attractive.

A girl goes through rapid body changes between the ages of twelve and fourteen years when breasts start developing, and between fourteen and eighteen they developfully. However, sometimes growth is stunted due to hormonal imbalance, congenital defects or deficiency of a nourishing diet. Wearing a shapely and tight brassiere since early developmental years is advisable in order to prevent sagging in later years. Remember, bras should not be too tight as this may cause cancer. During the development period girls should go in for activities like swimming, skipping, playing badminton or table-tennis, swinging or riding which gives vigorous exercise to the upper portion of the body.

Do not neglect Your Breasts
Examine your breasts regularly for lumps and bumps as this will enable you to detect any problems early and avoid complications

later. Lifted, well-rounded and shapely breasts of a female gives her an added attraction and such a bust symbolises youthful beauty. Shapeless, small, sluggish or over-developed breasts rob a woman of a streamlined figure. With the passing of youth, the busts droop, but if this happens in youthful days (due to sheer negligence it often happens with the majority of women in our country) early attention should be paid to avoid this defect.

Breast care is very important as it is among the erogeonous zones, and a feeding organ for a baby. If a woman's breasts sag and get flabby at an early age, it will fail to have any sexual attraction. A doctor had rightly said that there is no use of a breast which does not serve any purpose for a husband, nor to a baby.

Supporting Your Breasts
Breasts have no muscles of their own and are only held up by the pectoral muscles—the muscles of the chest on which they lie. Extra support can be given by wearing a good bra. Most of the support that a well-fitting bra gives to the breast should come from beneath and not from the straps. You can check this by slipping off the straps to see if the bra will stay in place without them. The back piece and the sides of a good bra should be in level with the front.

How to measure the Cups
If the bra cups are creased all over, then they are too big for your breast size. To find out the correct size of the bra cup, first measure around your rib cage under your breasts. Then measure around the fullest part of your bosom at the level of the nipple. The difference between the two measurements will give you the cup size.

How to choose a Bra
When choosing a bra for heavy breasts, make sure it has flat well-padded undercup wiring and wide elasticised straps that gives support to the centres of the breasts. Small breasts can be enhanced with the help of highly padded bras. Now the question is will the breasts sag, if you do not wear a bra? The sagging is due to the slackening of the supporting muscles, and is more possible if the breasts are heavy. Wearing a well-fitting bra will delay sagging for a little while. Always wear a good supporting bra during exercises, running, jogging and pregnancy. Exercising

neither reduces the size of heavy breasts, nor helps increase its size. Swimming is an excellent exercise for the bust shape and it strengthens the muscles. This is reason by swimmers have wonderfully shaped bustlines.

During pregnancy and the period of breast-feeding, the breasts become larger and elastic fibres in the skin tear, showing red irregular marks on the skin surface. By regular massage with a moisturising cream the elasticity of the skin is increased and the breast skin becomes soft and supple. Remember to remove bras at night. Underdeveloped breasts is a matter of great concern for women, but massaging with a nourishing cream is the only remedy.

Breast Care for Lactating Mothers

It is necessary to give supplements of vitamins or minerals to lactating mothers. In case the mother is healthy and the baby is not premature, there is no need to give vitamin supplements to the mother or to the baby at least three months after the delivery as breast milk supplies these in sufficient amounts to the baby. If the mother has any vitamin or mineral deficiencies or she is malnourished she may be required to take them. The mother may have a deficiency of vitamin B-12 if she is vegetarian. For a supply of Vitamin D, it is advisable for the mother to be in the sun for some time each day. In case the mother is deficient in Vitamin B-1, the baby can suffer serious symptoms. This problem is very rare but proper medical attention is very necessary. By improving the diet, vitamin deficiencies can be rectified. Mothers who are deficient in calcium should increase the intake of foods rich in calcium, like cabbage, lentils *(dals)*, milk, cheese and other milk products.

Care should be taken for breasts during lactation in the following ways:
 a) Keep your breasts and nipples clean and dry as this will prevent them from becoming sore and infected.
 b) Do not use soap to clean the nipples and areola since this may make them sore and cracked.
 c) Do not soak the nipples in water or let them remain moist as this will lead to cracking and infection of the nipples. Just wash the breasts and nipples with water during your daily bath.

d) The breasts may be cleaned with water to remove the traces of milk that might be sticking to them after a feed.

Crack and Fissure in the Nipple

The difference between a crack and a fissure is very little. A fissure is generally at the base of the nipple and is often very painful and may ooze blood. It may become infected if the baby has thrush in its mouth. In case a mother suffers from a fissure she may have to keep the baby off the breasts for a couple of days till the fissure heals. In case of a crack, a mother does not have to take the baby off the breast.

You must keep in mind the following precautions to prevent cracked or sore nipples:

a) Just wash your breasts with plain water and keep the nipples dry in between the feeds. If these are not kept dry, they tend to become sore. Therefore, do not soak nipples in water.
b) Do not clean the nipples with soap, as this leads to cracking.
c) If you experience the problem of leakage of milk, then absorb this leakage with a piece of clean cloth or cut a piece of cloth cut from a nappy, keep in the cups of your bra and change this as required.
d) Always wear a clean bra.
e) Clean your nipples after feeding.
f) Expose the nipples to air for some time every day.
g) Apply cream or oil to keep the nipples soft and supple. Do not use mustard oil, since it is irritating. Make sure to wash the cream or oil from the nipples before you breast-feed.
h) Apply cream or oil during the pregnancy, even though greasy material is produced during pregnancy which keeps the nipples supple.

How to treat a Cracked or Sore Nipple

Continue breast-feeding even if nipples are sore or cracked. Try to feed the baby from the less painful nipple first so that it does not hurt too much during feeding. By the time you have finished, the milk may start to drain from the other side and the breasts will become soft, allowing the baby to feed without suckling too hard. Express milk from your breasts to take tension away and prevent aggressive and painful suckling by the hungry baby.

Remember, pain can be reduced and healing promoted by paying attention to the way you breast-feed. Make sure that the areola is in the baby's mouth so that the baby cannot bite or chew at the nipples. Change your position every time you feed the baby so that the baby does not suckle at the nipple continuously in one position and make it more sore. Feed the child in such a position that the child is unable to pull the nipple. Do not remove the crusts of dried milk from a sore or a cracked nipple since this can worsen the situation. Occasionally blood oozing from the sore or cracked nipples may be swallowed by the baby, but it will not harm the baby in any way. If the problem is very severe then consult the doctor, who may suggest exposure to a sun-lamp and application of an antiseptic cream. Exposure of nipples to air for some time every day would help in the healing process.

The treatment of a fissure is the same as for a cracked or a sore nipple. Remember, the fissure may be considered more painful and you may have to use a nipple shield when you resume the baby on a breast-feed. Make sure that the nipple shield is clean.

Abdominoplasty—Body Contouring

A slim, supple figure is in vogue. Every woman is aware of the need to look and feel younger. Lax abdomens, wrinkled faces, sagging breasts, shapeless thighs are all causes of embarrassment to people who wish to look glamourous. Aesthetic surgery now offers new avenues to make you look better. If you have a lax, shapeless abdomen or the classical "fat aprons", you have a chance to get rid of it by a procedure commonly called Abdominoplasty or body contouring.

The vast majority of patients requiring abdominoplasty are females, but sometimes, males too suffer from it. The causes are:
a) Sudden weight loss.
b) Post-pregnancy.
c) Obesity and previous operations.

Abdominoplasty has become a common process. The main reasons for this are:
1) In modern society the emphasis is on youth and vigour.
2) A more liberal attitude towards sex.
3) Fashionable clothes that reveal the body.
4) More time spent in leisure and recreational activities.

The usual complaints are:
1) Marred skin, sagging and wrinkled.
2) A protruding abdomen.

Social and sexual activities are often limited by patients to avoid the embarrassment of exposing the abdomen. A vigorous exercise regimen helps to increase muscle tone but it will not improve the problem of excess skin nor will it correct the post-delivery pot belly. The ideal patient for abdominoplasty is:
1) A person normal in weight for his or her stature and height.
2) A woman who does not plan a further pregnancy.
3) A person ready to accept the inevitable surgical scar.

Abdominoplasty is primarily an aesthetic repair of the abdominal wall and is performed to correct deformities of skin, fat tissue and muscle. The abdominoplasty techniques are:
a) To permit resection of excess skin.
b) To close muscular separation and tighten their laxity
c) To leave a scar that can be sometimes hidden in the groin fold or can be hidden under a bikini suit.

Beware of taking aspirin-containing drugs ten days prior to surgery. Birth control pills and other hormones, when feasible, should be discontinued. A careful bath with medicated soap for two days before surgery is advised. The choice of surgical technique depends upon the anatomic deformity in individual cases.

The skin incision begins just inside the pubic hairline and curves gently to the groin skin crease. The skin flap alongwith the fatty layer, is separated from the deeper muscles up to the umbilical level. The excess of skin and fatty tissues are excised after locating the umbilicus at the desired level. Post-operative pain and discomfort is usually moderate and limits activities for 2 to 3 days. The patient is allowed to move after the fifth day. All sutures are removed within 10 to 15 days and normal activities are resumed slowly. Vigorous activities like swimming, running and playing should be avoided for 6 to 8 weeks. Remember, abdominoplasty should be done by an experienced surgeon only.

10

COMMON CONDITIONS OF GENITALIA

Scabies, Warts, Herpes, Candidiasis (or Moniliasis), Phimosis and Aids Virus are some of the common conditions of the genitalia.

Genital Scabies
Quite often lesions of scabies may be seen on the genitals. Apart from intense nocturnal itching, the lesions are observed as papules on the prepuce, glans and shaft of the pens and scrotum with the burrow tract seen as a thin, black irregular line on top. Very often, scratching by the patient removes the top, leaving a small shallow ulcer and subsequent crusting. Female genitalia are rarely affected by this condition.

Genital Warts
Like anywhere else on the body, surface warts can also occur on genitalia. Genital warts are usually transmitted by sexual contact, though auto-inoculation from the hands may sometimes occur. They can occur in both sexes and are usually located on the moist surface of the genitalia. They start as minute reddish swellings and grow into grouped pedunculated lesions. The genital warts usually respond to local applications of 20 per cent podophyllin in tincture benzoinco. While applying this agent, the surrounding normal area has to be protected with petroleum jelly.
    (Remember to consult your doctor before any treatment.)

Genital Herpes
This is caused by a different strain of the same virus, caught by having sex with someone who has herpes. It is common in young people. Groups of little blisters appear on the genital area, thighs and buttocks. They are painful, tender and highly infectious. The

first infection is the worst with swollen glands and a temperature. The blisters crust over and clear in seven to ten days. The virus becomes dormant but may cause repeated attacks. When coping with genital herpes, the virus hidden in the nerves cannot be killed. Anti-viral creams and lotions, used immediately, may shorten an attack. Warm salt water baths and pain-killers (Aspirin and Paracetamol as recommended by the doctor) make you more comfortable during an attack. All attacks of genital herpes are infectious. Avoid having sex during an attack, but once the scabs have disappeared, you can have it again. Condoms lessen the risk of infection. Genital herpes is in the news and people have been frightended by speculations in the press. Repeated herpes can be a big problem, but mostly people have a single mild attack. Frequent attacks of genital herpes play havoc with your sex life, but new vaccines and anti-viral drugs are being developing in our country to combat this infectious disease. Worry and depression, poor general health, lack of sleep and an unhealthy diet may reduce your resistance to infection. An attack of genital herpes in pregnancy is very serious as an infected mother can pass on the infection to her baby and so she may need to be delivered by a Caesarean section.

Candidiasis or Moniliasis
This is caused by an yeast called Candida. Genital infection is common in uncircumcised males. It usually presents as radial fissures on the prepucial margin. The inner surface of the prepuce becomes edematous and macerated and shows white flakes. Retraction of the prepuce is difficult and painful and the glans penis is inflamed. In women, candidiasis may not have any symptom. It is very important to note that a large number of normal females in the reproductive age group normally have candida as normal flora of the vagina. Certain factors like the state of pregnancy, diabetes, administration of broad spectrum antibiotics and steroids and also the use of contraceptive pills appear to cause the organism to produce the clinical condition. In women, it produces a white vaginal discharge with intense irritation. There may also be burning micturition.

The treatment consists of the application of anti-fungal preparations to all skin and mucosal surfaces involved to eliminate the fungus while preventing reinfection from the sex partner. Any causative factor mentioned above should be

Common Conditions of Genitalia

investigated and suitable treatment with the consultation of your doctor instituted. The anti-fungal preparations available include nystation (Mycostatin), micanazole (Dactarin), clotrimazole (Clomazole, Imidil) which can be used locally as creams in both males and females. In addition, nystation and clotrimazole can also be used as tablets inserted intravaginally daily for two weeks and six days respectively in females.

Phimosis and Aids Virus

This refers to a condition in males in which the prepucial opening (formed by the foreskin covering the terminal part of the penis—the glans penis) of the male organ is narrow. Though it can result from chronic or acute infection of the inner lining of the prepuce, more commonly it is congenital.

The Aids virus depresses immunity, increasing the risk of common and rare infections and rare cancers. It may be transmitted hetero sexually or by infected blood products but use of condoms reduces the risk.

Tumours of the Skin

(This chapter has been compiled with the help of Skin Specialist Dr. Jitender Arora.)

The excessive exposure of the skin to sunrays can lead to cancer of the skin. Thus sunbathing, the latest health trend, needs proper precautions. The sunlight, particularly during its peak four hours, can lead to solar keratosis, tumours, nevi, basal and squamous cell carcinoma and the melanomas. So the best precautionary measure is shelter from the sun and protective sunscreen lotions or creams while sunbathing, though proper clothing is equally important.

Benign Tumours

These are the seborrhoeic warts, and consist of a benign growth of epithelium, a pigmented velvety, warty surface. They are relatively more common, both on covered and uncovered surfaces. These can also be mistaken for melanomas of cutaneous neoplasma.

Nevi

The nevus cells and nevi are almost always benign and everybody may have it at one stage of life or the other. They usually appear in children and are fibrosed during old age. The pigmented congenital nevi presents a greater tendency to form melanoma. They should be surgically removed when they appear. The junctional nevi has nevus cells on both sides of the epidermal junction and consists of clear nevus cells alongwith some melanin. If it grows rapidly, darkens or bleeds, surgical consultation becomes essential. Likewise, other nevi are compound nevi, blue nevi, and epithelial nevi.

Premalignant Tumours

The premalignant tumours are the borderline stage. So if controlled at this stage they can be cured. The solar keratoses are flesh-coloured and coarse to touch. But if they degenerate, they become the squamous cell carcinoma. In people with fair complexions, they occur mostly on the exposed parts. Nonactinic keratoses occur due to arsenic exposures. The cells are typical and similar to those of squamous cell epitheliomas, but these changes are well contained by an intact epidermal-dermal junction.

Malignant Tumours

Squamous cell carcinoma occurs on the exposed parts of such people who sunburn easily and tan poorly. They may arise out of actinic or solar keratoses, and attain a diameter of one centimetre just within two weeks. The lesions are small, red, conical, hard nodules which have a quick tendency to ulcerate. Metastasis may occur early. The treatment of choice is surgical excision and even X-ray radiation is useful.

The basal cell carcinoma also occurs mostly on the exposed parts, but these lesions grow very slowly and attain a size of 1 cm after about a year. The appearance is waxy and the metastasis almost never occur. The neglected lesions may ulcerate and produce great destruction of even vital organs. The treatment is almost the same as in squamous cell carcinoma.

Paget's disease may occur around the nipple because of the manifestation of apocrine sweat gland carcinoma, and may also occur in the genitalia. The malignant melanoma vary from macule to nodule with a surprising play of colours from flesh tints to pitch black, and a frequent mixture of white, blue, purple and red. The border tends to be irregular and the growth may be rapid. The treatment consists of wide surgical excision with lymphnodes. As reports confirm out of three human cancer cases,

Common Conditions of Genitalia

one is a case of skin cancer while one out of a hundred is a melanoma.

Difference between Skin Cancer and Tumours

A skin tumour is caused by excessive exposure to sunrays and in case it is not treated in time, may lead to skin cancer. Also avoid excess exposure to X-rays. Keratosis is another form of skin cancer in old age when numerous scaly patches appear on the scalp and other areas, such as the face, ear and back of the hands. Fleshy rapidly-growing lumps of bumps in the skin may spread to the other parts of the body and should be dealt with immediately. Skin cancer rarely spreads to the rest of the body but needs to be removed by an experienced surgeon by "Radiotherapy", "Surgery" and "Cryotherapy" (liquid nitrogen can be used to kill cancer cells by freezing). The commonest skin cancer is Rodent Ulcer.

Try to get skin cancer diagnosed at the earliest. It is easier to treat in early stages. Get it treated by an experienced doctor. There are several types of skin lightening creams or bleaching creams available in the market and they all contain a chemical called Hydroquinone which interferes with the production of melanin. These creams cannot lighten the post-inflammatory pigmentation which is the common cause of brown patches though they can lighten the normal skin, birthmarks and freckles. It is generally very irritating to the skin and causes inflammation with more darkening of the skin, or blotchy discoloration. In case of itching or redness, stop using bleaching creams immediately. Use of hydroquinone especially in high concentration (5 per cent and above) preparations sometimes damage the underlying tissues, leaving black lumps and cysts. It is better to use 2 per cent hydroquinone creams unless advised otherwise by a dermatologist. Monobenzyl ether of hydroquinone may contaminate bleaching creams and can cause permanent colour loss.

Cystitis

Are you married?
Do You have burning sensation on the skin around the vagina whenever passing urine?
Do you experience continuous aching, inflammation and severe pain when having sexual intercourse?
These may be the signs of cystitis.

Generally, clinics are filled with women patients suffering from skin complaints (apart from gynaecological problems). The problem is that the female anatomy was designed by God—who, we must assume was a man and didn't understand the trouble he was causing! It could be anyone, perhaps, your cousin, who faces painful and embarrassing conditions like the frequent urge to rush to the toilet, the feeling of not quite being able to empty the urinary bladder, a burning sensation on urination (called micturition), backache, feverishness and sometimes blood in the urine (called haematuria). In a woman's life, there are three main phases when she is most likely to suffer from cystitis: at the beginning of her sex life, after childbirth or surgery, or with menopause.

Before going ahead, here are some basic details. The word 'cystitis' means bladder (cystis) and inflammation (itis). But more often than being just a bladder inflammation, it is the urethra, the short outlet tube from the bladder, which gets severely affected. The urethra generally suffers physical damage during sexual intercourse, rape, surgery, childbirth, menopause or even a clumsy pelvic examination. Or an irritant to blame is a soap, deodorant, antiseptic or contraceptive cream. Sometimes an infection to the vagina is to blame and sometimes the condition is aggravated by a blocked or tight urethra. Human bodily metabolism involves the regular intake of essentials such as the food we eat and the air we breathe and regular discharge of waste products from the body. These are processed through the urinary tract which comprises the kidneys, the ureters, bladder and urethra. It is the job of the kidneys to filter the blood and to excrete much of these wastes in the form of urine. An adult normally has two bean-shaped kidneys about 10 cm long and each weighing between 120 and 180 gm. About 1,200 ml blood flows through the kidneys each minute, filling and purifying the entire bloodstream in about five minutes. The waste product urine is produced at a rate of about one millilitre per minute and the rest of the fluid containing substances such as salts and sugars are returned to the body. The urine is removed from the kidney by ureters, the two thin tubes, and are stored temporarily in the bladder, a thin walled muscular sac with a mucous lining. The storage capacity of the bladder is roughly a pint (0.56 litre). In infants, the bladder automatically empties as soon as the volume of urine in the bladder reaches a certain level. But as children are trained, they learn to control this action. The causes of cystitis range from sexual, dietary, environmental and the physiological to psychological. The majority of sufferers fall into three main groups: first, those whose cystitis coincide with the onset of active sexual life where symptoms appear after love-making. The second group consists of middle-aged women whose symptoms can be traced back to physical damage caused by a difficult labour, catheterisation, hysterectomy or even a careless internal medical examination. The third group comprises those whose symptoms follow the menopause when the level of the female hormone oestrogen drops and the vagina and urethra become dry and less pliable. Many of these cases are linked with the onset of sexual activity. This complaint not only mars the enjoyment of sexual encounters but also practically ruins marriages. A relationship with a woman frigid with pain and the fear of causing further unbearable pain, requires a very great deal of mutual understanding. Treatment by some good doctor is essential. The female urethra is hardly one inch long and is very close to and similar to the vagina—both organs have exactly the same mucous lining, making them susceptible to the same infections and changes in hormone levels. The outlet of the female urethra is usually situated next to the outlet of the vagina. On the other side of the vagina is the anus which is also a potential source of infection. It is the close proximity of these three outlets that underlies many cases of cystitis. Bacteria occurring in this part of the body (called the perineum) can enter the urethra and rapidly multiply in its warm, moist environment, causing inflammation and ultimately, burning pain. There are certain other complications causing this problem such as when the outlet of the urethra sometimes may be found just inside the vagina or when during love-making it may open temporarily into the vagina swollen with sexual excitement. As a cosmetologist, I will suggest that hygiene of the affected area is essential. The infection is probably due to higher sexual activity among pill users. Avoid use of contraceptives, creams and jellies (containing chemicals) which, in sensitive women, may further irritate the condition thus triggering cystitis-type symptoms. Douches, deodorants, pessaries, and even soaps contain chemicals which may irritate a sensitive skin.

Avoid use of the type of food that might set off allergic reactions. The urinary symptoms in some women are related to irritants in foods, alcohol, toiletries and even to nylon underwear which sometimes cause allergy. Beware of bubble baths which not only contain chemicals that may irritate, but which also lower surface tension and allow soapy water and bacteria to penetrate higher into the vagina than ordinary bath water does. Soap, deodorants, powders, nylon underwear—which feels beautifully silky when dry but, when damp, acts on the skin like fine sandpapers—are avoidable. Detergents not properly rinsed out of underwear during washing cause further harm to the cystitis sufferer. Be sure to avoid nylon underwear in any season.

Vaginal thrush, herpes genitalis, trichomonas vaginalis are some of conditions which may produce similar symptoms. So it is better to consult a doctor who will conduct a detailed examination of the affected region around the vagina. He will conduct an internal examination with a cotton swab. A urine sample will be taken for further investigations. X-rays will probably be recommended for women with recurrent infections. The treatment of drug therapy includes use of antibiotics (Ampicillin, Co-trimoxazole, Sulphonamides, Nitrofurantoin, Steptomycin, Nalidixic acid, Tetracyclines). Hormonal therapy, surgery, dilatation, urethrotomy, urethroplasty, catheterisation are some of the treatments for which a consultation of a doctor is necessary. Personal hygiene, wearing cotton underwear, drinking the maximum amount of water, washing your perineum from front to back after each time you pass urine, are some easy ways to cure cystitis.

All You Wanted To Know About

Rs. 50/- each

Parapsychology/Spiritual Sciences

- ....2396 1 Spiritual Healing
- ....2395 3 Spirituality
- ....2297 3 Nostradamus
- ....2274 4 Dowsing
- ....2367 8 Psychic Development
- ....2350 3 Aura
- ....2271 x Hypnosis

Personal Transformation

- ....2391 0 Relaxation
- ....2388 0 Happiness
- ....2325 2 Hatha Yoga
- ....2326 0 Kriya Yoga
- ....2347 3 Meditation
- ....2327 9 Kundalini
- ....2324 4 Chakras and Nadis
- ....2233 7 Reiki
- ....2354 6 Mantras

Self-Understanding

- ....2336 8 Tarot
- ....2351 1 Dreams
- ....2337 6 Chinese Astrology
- ....2328 7 Sun Signs
- ....2194 2 Astrology
- ....2196 9 Graphology
- ....2198 5 Palmistry
- ....2195 0 Gems
- ....2197 7 Numerology

Self-Help & Success

- ....2394 5 Self Motivation
- ....2392 9 Relationships
- ....2387 2 Secrets of Magic
- ....2393 7 As a Man Thinketh
- ....2378 3 Vedic Mathematics
- ....2348 1 Stress & Anger
- ....2349 x Secret of Success
- ....2275 2 Feng Shui
- ....2323 6 I Ching
- ....2199 3 Vastushastra
- ....2273 6 Increasing Memory Power

Alternative Medicine

- ....2308 7 Yoga for Health and Happiness
- ....2368 6 Sun Therapy
- ....2276 0 Magnetotherapy

All You Wanted To Know About

Rs.50/- each

....2301 5	Acupressure in Daily Life	
....2272 8	Aromatherapy	
....2232 9	Yoga	
....2231 0	Healing Powers of Water	

Law for the Layman

....2399 6	Filing Income Tax Returns
....2400 3	Income Tax
....2397 x	Buy, Rent, Sell Property
....2398 8	How to prepare your own Will

Health

....2386 4	Family Planning
....2352 x	Fitness
....2353 8	Hair Care
....2355 4	Weight Reduction
....2305 8	Kidney Stones
....2307 4	Typhoid
....2303 1	First Aid
....2306 6	Menstrual Irregularities
....2300 7	Menopause
....2302 3	Chronic Bronchitis
....2335 x	Acne
....2299 x	Diarrhoea
....2304 x	HIV and AIDS
....2222 1	Anxiety
....2224 8	Diabetes
....2226 4	Headache
....2227 2	Heart Attack
....2225 6	Hepatitis
....2229 9	Knee Joint Pain
....2228 0	Hypertension
....2230 2	Nutrition
....2223 x	Constipation

The English Language

....2217 5	Vocabulary & Usage
....2215 9	Proficiency in English
....2213 2	Business English
....2214 0	English Grammar
....2216 7	Spoken English
....2212 4	Letter Writing

Baby Names

....2329 5	Namkaran: Name for Baby Boys
....2298 1	Namkaran: Name for Baby Girls
....2270 1	Baby Names: For the New Millennium
....2269 8	Baby Names: From the Scriptures